Clean Eating:

The Essential Healthy Eating Bundle For Lasting Weight Loss- Change Your Diet, Change Your Health, Change Your Life!

I0409302

Clean Eating

Ketogenic Diet

Lean Diet

Clean Eating:

The Simple & Amazing Guide to Improve Your Health, Lose Weight & Feel Great Without Dieting!

Introduction

Thank you for purchasing the book, 'Clean Eating: The Simple & Amazing Guide to Improve Your Health, Lose Weight & Feel Great without Dieting!'

It is true that you may have had diets that you have not been able to stick to. You may also have had a diet that requires you to drink only fruit juices! You may have tried numerous diets like the Paleo diet and may have also tried to dip cotton balls into the juice in order to lose weight!

But, you may have found that you have not changed at all. The weight you have been trying to shed has clung to you like a leech. You have lost all the energy and stamina you used to have too! The glow on your face does not exist anymore and when you look at yourself in the mirror you wonder what has happened to you. It is true that you lost all the extra pounds in your body initially, but what happened afterwards? They came right back into your body! What on earth happened to you?

There is only one reason behind this and that is because you have unhealthy eating habits. It is because of this reason that you did not get rid of the fat that has found a home for itself in your body. Through this book, you will be able to understand the mistakes you have been making while on a diet and how you can rectify those mistakes. You will be given a diet that will be like no other – a diet that will keep you healthy and wait for it, help you lose weight too!

At this point, you may already be well-versed in the concept of clean eating. Or you may be wondering, "What exactly is this diet that I have heard so much about?" Imagine the lifestyle that our ancestors led. They tended the earth and relied on its fruits to sustain them. Modern grocery stores did not even exist until 1916. The idea of a self-service grocery store was put in motion by Clarence Saunders, founder of the Piggly Wiggly chain. Saunders was awarded multiple patents for his innovations regarding convenience at the time.

In the beginning, this revolutionary idea was a lucrative and helpful addition to many communities. These stores opened jobs and increased the demand of local products from businesses and farms. But during the course of the past century, the focus has seemed to shift from the concern of accessibility to profit at the expense of public health. Unfortunately, because of the exponential growth and demand of big box stores, the consumer often suffers from some nasty side effects. The mass production food industry has systematically reduced the quality of their product in favor of cheaper and less healthful alternatives.

The concept of clean eating is really not so far-fetched. It is simply the mentality that nature knows best and that the body needs natural food as fuel to function efficiently. It is the decision to purchase and consume only whole foods. That is, food that is free from processes such as the refining of grains and sugars, additions of artificial additives, colors and preservatives, and the application of pesticides.

But first, before getting too deep into forming clean eating habits, let us touch on the meaning of the word 'diet'. Dieting is not necessarily synonymous to fasting. Dieting in the context of this book is the kinds of food you eat. It is the same context used when people refer to things like the ketogenic diet, paleo diet, and etc. In order to form good clean eating habits, you must change and develop a clean eating lifestyle. Clean eating, losing weight, and staying fit is not a one and done deal. It is a whole lifestyle that you must adapt in order to achieve the body and health level that you want in life.

I hope you enjoy the book and begin your journey on a new path towards health! Thank you.

Chapter 1: Clean Eating 101

There are numerous diets that you may have tried in order to get rid of all the fat that has settled in your body. You may have noticed that the diets have not done much when it came to help you become healthier. Yes, you did lose weight initially, but do you have the stamina that you once had? Did you find yourself healthier than before? You may not have it anymore and this is due to the fact that you do not have healthy eating habits. It is for this very reason that you will need to learn a little more about what clean eating is in order to get rid of the unwanted fat in your body.

You will find yourself helpless irrespective of whether or not you exercise or spend an exorbitant amount of money on fruits and vegetables that are not available at home if you do not eat right! Heath has all come down to clean eating. It has become a trend and you will find people at work or in the neighborhood discussing clean eating and how great it has bee n for them. But, like every other trend, this one has its own misconceptions too! There are certain people who believe that kiwi in New Zealand is the best for health when it comes to obtaining Vitamin C. This is great news for the people living in New Zealand. What about the people living in the other parts of the world? If you go to a gym, the trainer there will tell you what it is that you need to do in order to lose weight. They will ask you to buy whey protein shakes and you will rush to the nearest supermarket to do the same! There are people all over the world who would love to mislead you. This is because of the fact that they believe that the diet that has helped them will help the rest of the world! However, often at times these diets always leave people feeling malnourished and unhealthy.

Let us consider that you have walked into a diner and have ordered their Big Juicy Burger! This is a delicacy is it not – the lovely buns, with the patty and the layers of vegetables. It does sound healthy to you does it not? Well, that is where you are wrong! The food that is used to make the burger has been produced industrially implying that it is full of fat, which will leave you with more calories that you had accounted for!

What does this mean for you then? Do you have the basic picture of what clean eating is? It means that you have to consume food that is whole, natural and something that does not pour itself out of the different containers in the supermarkets. It is always good to consume food that comes from gardens since they have the best nutrients! This is what clean eating is all about. Yes, it is that simple! This is a concept that has emerged in the late 1970s when people were craving to find their health!

I mentioned earlier that there were misconceptions about clean eating. Let us clear those out shall we?

The myths of clean eating

It is a diet

Well, let me stop you right there. When you look at the honest meaning of the word diet, you will be shocked or slightly guilty. A diet is a plan that any human being will willingly follow for a month or two in order to lose all the unwanted fat in his or her body. What happens after? You will be sick of the fact that you are starving yourself when you can consume whatever food you love since you have lost enough weight. These diets are short-term solutions and leave you unhappy since they require that you throw out all the snacks in your house! Have you seen the show on Modern Family where Cameron decides to go on a Juice Fast and gets rid of every single item he loves to eat? You may be forced to do that too. Instead of going through all this pain, it is best for you to start eating clean! You will be able to keep yourself healthy and will also find yourself feeling positive about life. You would not be a crabby person like Cameron was when he was on the diet.

A restriction on intake of calories

When you begin to eat in a clean manner, you will be able to fill your body with all the nutrients you need. You will find yourself energetic and happy no matter what the situation may be. Any requirement that your metabolism has will have been met if you start eating clean. You will never have to worry about the numerous calories you may be consuming in the process since they are used up by your body in the right way.

Higher frequency of meals

There are people all over the world who will tell you different things. Some may ask you to consume meals thrice a day while some may say that you will need to consume meals six times or maybe even ten times a day. What they have forgotten is that you will need to focus on the content of the meal and not on the number of times you consume a meal. You could consume small portions every day but there is no point in eating chips, cereal or even chocolate! This is because of the fact that your health will go for a toss if you do this! You have to be careful of what you eat. If you consume all the right amount of food, you will find that your weight has begun to stabilize itself and your energy levels have gone up! You will be allowed to eat whenever you want and how much ever you want as long as you choose to eat clean.

Deprivation

When you begin to eat clean, you do not have to stop consuming the food that you love. You will only be looking for alternatives that are healthier. Now, if you are someone who loves potato wedges and fries, all you have to do is bake them instead of frying them in oil! Ensure that the desserts you consume are made using flour that is healthy for your body. Try to make any form of fast food at home instead of consuming that from any diner near your house! If you want to give in to comfort food, all you have to do is compensate for that food with a healthier meal during the day! You could consume a huge chunk of a blueberry cake with one wholesome meal and you would be giving yourself the nutrition that you need.

Chapter 2: Understanding The Principles of Clean Eating

You have now gathered a decent idea on what clean eating is all about, so let us look at a few principles that will help you with eating healthy. You will need to keep these principles in mind before you jump on board with clean eating.

Natural food over processed food

If you purchase food from the supermarket and find that you are picking up products that come out of a bag, can, or even a box, remind yourself that these foods are definitely processed. However, you may think to yourself that the frozen vegetables are not processed, so why choose frozen vegetables instead of fresh produce? When you consume fresh food, you will be able to ensure that you have great health for a very long time. It is always good to consume fresh and crisp food if you are looking at keeping yourself healthy. If you find that you are feeling good on the inside it will reflect on the outside.

Prefer unrefined food

This is a fact that everybody needs to remember! Make sure that you consume your share of wheat, rice, barley, millets and quinoa whenever you can! It is always good to consume food that gives you protein – make sure that the food is not refined! If you love sweetened food, make sure that you consume maple syrup or even honey instead of downing spoons of sugar. Always choose these foods over boxed foods since they are the best for your health.

Always consume a balanced meal

When you are preparing a meal for yourself, you have to ensure that you have not broken the contents of the meal down. Do not tell yourself that you need proteins and carbohydrates right before a workout since this does not help your body. You will have to include every nutrient that you need in one meal a day! You will have to avoid depriving your body of these nutrients simply because of a certain a schedule or diet you used to follow.

Keep an eye on sugar and fat

The fat we are discussing about here is trans-fat which is extremely and terribly bad for your body. These fats find their homes in your arteries and conveniently block them causing millions of heart diseases. If you consume salt and sugar in the right amounts you would not be harming your body. But, too much of these ingredients would only lead to numerous health issues that you would never want to be associated with ever!

Always understand your body's needs

Every human is different from the next. The way your body is built is definitely different from the way mine is built. Therefore, it is difficult to tell you to stick to a diet that I may have tried since that may not work for you! You have to consume three meals a day and will need to ensure that you have included every group of food into those meals. The minute you begin to skip meals, your body begins to starve itself and will use up the fat in your body. This is good news but what you have forgotten is that the next time you eat food, it all gets stored as fat in your body! You could also consume healthy snacks in between if that is what your body needs! Make sure that you consume a salad or fruit.

Always exercise!

This is something that you will definitely need to do. You will not have to work out in the gym for hours together. You just need to ensure that you continue to move. If you are watching the television and the advertisements have begun, go for a walk around the living room. Make sure that you incorporate as much exercise as possible. There are countless apps for smart phones and other short 5 minute workout programs you can include in your day to day life.

Always shop smart

When you have entered the supermarket, what aisle do you walk up to first? You will walk up to the aisles where you have seen the numerous boxes with all the lovely food stored in them. You put the fresh produce out of your mind and continue to shop for these packaged items! The next time you enter a supermarket, walk up to the fresh produce first and pick the ingredients you need before you walk down the other aisles.

No added sugar

This is a principle that every human being has to follow! You will need to stop consuming excessive amounts of sugar. You will only be feeding your body with calories that do nothing to keep you healthy. Food in the natural form contains the required amounts of sugar. You could consume fruits or even a few vegetables to obtain the sugar you want. Ensure that you do not consume cold fruit juices or soda since they are filled to their brim with sugar. Just take a look at the amount of sugar in a can of soda. You will find yourself loving natural foods when you have warmed up to the idea mentioned above. You may find that not consuming as much sugar as normal will decrease your energy levels, but that is okay! The reason why is that your body will need to go through a temporary transitional period in which your body is not so heavily reliant on artificial energy through the means of consuming sugar. Once this transitional period has passed, you will have constant real and healthy energy!

Drink lots of water

You have been told that you need to consume close to eight or ten glasses of water and this is with great reason. There are reasons behind this. The first is that you have to keep your body hydrated since your muscles will be able to respond faster and you will also be able to continue to the work out with ease. The second is that the organs in your body will begin to function in the normal way. The final reason is that you always confuse your thirst with hunger!

Always sit down to eat

Every human being has become very busy these days. They do not have the time to sit down and consume their meal since they are always rushing out of the house in order to get to work on time. Other times you consume your dinner in front of the television. You will find that you will consume too much food that may also include junk. You have to stop this and will need to start making sure that you make every meal a special affair. You will need to set the table out and also ensure that you serve each morsel with care. You could invite friends over and also have your family sitting with you at the table. You will find that you will be able to consume a great home cooked meal.

Are you scared of the flour used in desserts?

You could definitely eat that lovely pastry, the mouthwatering pie, and the lovely cake just by substituting the flour with a healthier version of the flour! You could definitely use millet flour or even almond flour instead of the all – purpose flour when you are baking at home. You will find that the final product is not that different from the original recipe and the advantage here is that you will be able to eat your favorite food in its healthiest form.

Always consume food you understand

When you are looking at the boxes you have purchased, have you made the effort to read the list of ingredients that have been mentioned at the back of the box? Do you understand every ingredient that has been mentioned? Are there certain items that you cannot read at all? Can you pronounce every ingredient? It is best if you do not consume such processed foods filled with preservatives. You could always choose to stick to food that you have a great knowledge of. If you find that the food you want to eat comes in a box, you will need to chuck it. Always try to use food that you can read and pronounce. The food could be exotic but this does not mean it is good for your health. Always consume whole food!

Nutrition is more important than calories

Every person in the world has become very conscious of the food that he or she consumes. It is true that people need to control their caloric intake, but this does not mean they cut it out of their diet. The calories are needed by your body in order to help it function. You need to focus on the nutritional value of the food you consume and stop worrying about the calories. Your body is more intelligent than you know and can always differentiate between good and bad calories.

Chapter 3: Why Choose the Clean Eating Lifestyle?

Eating a clean and unprocessed diet is first and foremost for your overall health. Weight loss is just an added bonus. You must enter into this decision with the mentality that you are doing this for the big picture because getting into a state of better health is paramount. We come equipped with only one ephemeral vessel to carry us throughout our years and that cliché' phrase, "You are what you eat" remains true. The food we choose fuels these wondrous machines of ours. In order to best care for ourselves and ensure a long and healthy life, we must become more mindful of our eating habits.

We have discussed the many benefits of what I call a lifestyle because it requires you to change your outlook and not just your grocery list. Now, we will touch on the results you will experience by using this knowledge over any fad diet. Dr. Layne Norton claims that most diets fail due to lack of consistency and an inability to adapt the lifestyle necessary for continuance on your path. His research has also found that within a year, 80% of dieters will gain back the weight they had lost and a quarter of those eventually gain more weight. This yo-yo effect of crash dieting is extremely detrimental to your health, motivation and progress.

Adopting a clean lifestyle encourages the intake of fruits, vegetables, lean meats, nuts, seeds, healthy grains and fats. It also promotes exercise and restricts additives and preservatives commonly found in most processed foods. Chowing down on nuts like almonds or walnuts, for example, can lower your cholesterol and thereby greatly reducing the risk of heart disease. These, as well as olive oil, avocados, and fatty fish like salmon, all have something in common. They contain unsaturated fats. Monounsaturated and polyunsaturated fats – including the famed omega 3 and omega 6 – are essential fatty acids that your body can't make on its own.

Whole grain fiber and protein from nuts, legumes and lean meats are digested slowly and serve as a sustainable energy source that will keep you fuller for longer periods of time. And among other benefits, plant foods contain the high probiotic and enzyme content essential for a healthy intestinal ecology. Thriving gut flora enables proper nutrient absorption and disposal of waste.

A study published in the British Journal of Health Psychology suggested that young adults who observed a clean eating lifestyle experienced a greater "flourishing", meaning they were happier, more positive, creative, and curious. Another study, found in the Australian and New Zealand Journal of Psychiatry, has found a correlation in patients who experienced psychosis and their intake of fruits and vegetables. There are countless other social experiments and studies which point to an overall feeling of happiness and tranquility associated with clean eating habits. When we understand what our bodies need to thrive and provide them with such they will in turn take care of us!

Have you ever had trouble falling asleep or staying asleep? Can you not seem to relax or clear your mind? Well, you are not alone. Over 50 million Americans claim they do not get enough sleep. Modifying your diet to include fish such as salmon, halibut, and tuna can boost vitamin B which is needed to make Melatonin, the sleep-inducing hormone. I would bet that you never thought of carb loading to induce sleep, either. Well, in one study conducted by the American Journal of Clinical Nutrition, participants who consumed high glycemic index (GI) jasmine rice at dinner fell asleep faster than those who had a meal prepared with lower GI long-grain rice. This could be attributed to the greater amount of insulin which jump started the production of tryptophan, another sleep-inducing chemical.

Whatever your reason for taking up the cause of caring for your body might be, whether it's weight loss, better sleep, improved brain and gut health, immune boost, high cholesterol, cancer treatment, or even a general state of happiness and well-being, the importance of eating for your health is obvious and the time is now.

Chapter 4: The Negative Effects of Processed Foods

An epidemic is currently sweeping this nation with over half of Americans classified as either overweight or obese. Ranking among the lowest of industrialized nations in terms of life expectancy, Americans spend on average about $1,200 each year on fast food. Monetary concerns aside, the negative health effects of processed foods are staggering. Foods can be considered processed through a number of alterations ranging from chemical fillers to just adding heat during cooking. Observing a clean eating lifestyle, you would want to stay as close to the foods whole and natural state as possible. The exception would be a process - such as cooking or dehydrating at home - that doesn't add harmful chemicals into the mix. When foods start receiving chemical fillers, additives, and preservatives that is when we cross over into more dangerous territory. Junk foods are comprised of anything that contain hydrogenated fats, chemicals, nitrates, preservatives, or a high refined sugar content. These processed options have something in common; the cost of digesting, absorbing, and eliminating these non-foods is far greater than any nutritional and caloric benefit they may offer.

The ancient art of food preservation such as canning, salting, fermentation, and sun-drying are almost extinct in the modern world of mass production. Today, there are thousands of additives and chemicals used by food companies. Not all of which are bad such as the addition of calcium or vitamins. Many of these, however, can wreak havoc on our bodies.

Nitrates are chemicals used to preserve and cure certain meats and have been associated with cancer, asthma, nausea, and headaches. Sulfur dioxide is another toxic preservative that is used in dried fruit and molasses and also prevents brown spots on peeled fresh food like apples. The application of this chemical snuffs out the vitamin B content of these foods and often hides telltale signs of inferior produce. When you hear that antioxidants may be used to preserve certain foods, you would probably think, "Great! Antioxidants are good for the body, right?" Well, not always. Antioxidants such as BHA (butylated hydroxyanisole) and BHA (butylated hydroxytoluene) are two of the most controversial and widely used examples. The results of animal testing were so disturbing, that a number of countries have significantly restricted their use or banned them altogether. Some scientists have found correlations between these additives and hyperactivity disorder, behavioral problems, allergic reactions, cancer, and neurological damage. Despite these findings, the United States has not put any limitations on companies who use these antioxidants. The prevalence of BHA and BHT in food products has actually increased in the U.S.

Artificial food dyes are another additive that food companies use in everything from orange rinds, to chicken feed in order to produce a more yellow yolk. Blue #1 was found to cause kidney tumors in mice, according to an unpublished study concerning the effects of dyes on animal subjects. Blue #2, commonly found in colored beverages, candies, and pet food was found to significantly increase the incidence of brain gliomas and other tumors in male rats. Citrus red #2 is the dye used to enhance the color of orange skins and also caused tumors in rodents. Recognized in 1990 as a thyroid carcinogen, red #3 is added to sausage casings, maraschino cherries, and candies. Red #40 is widely consumed and has been said to accelerate immune system tumors in mice. Found in baked goods, dessert powders, candies, cereals, and cosmetics, "Allura Red" has also been linked to hyperactivity in children. Yellow #5 and yellow #6 have both been studied in connection with hypersensitivity and hyperactivity in children and adrenal tumors in rodents. These two are commonly found in products such as gelatin desserts, candies, soda, and cosmetics.

With the frighteningly high prevalence of Autism and hyperactivity disorders observed in American children recently, one cannot help but to connect the dots from the harmful chemicals added to food during processing to an exponential increase in these diseases. According to the CDC as of 2011, approximately 11% of children – 6.4 million – have been diagnosed with ADHD. The percentage of children with a hyperactivity diagnosis has significantly increased from 7.8% in 2003. Rates of ADHD diagnoses increased on an average of 3% per year from 1997-2006 and approximately 5% per year from 2003-2011. As well as these hyperactivity disorders, Autism spectrum disorders have consistently been on the rise parallel with increased use of additives in mass produced foods. Records from the CDC have shown that ASD is on the rise from 1 in 150 in 2000 to 1 in 68 as of 2012. Considering the calculation of growth, diagnoses have likely soared to 1 in 50 or less in 2015.

Artificial sweeteners have been the subject of much scrutiny over the years. New alternatives come and go. Most notably, saccharine and aspartame. Saccharine was found to increase the incidence of bladder cancer in animals and companies that still use this product have been required to include warning information on the label. Aspartame is one of the most common artificial sweetener used today. Countless studies have been conducted about the safety of aspartame and most were inconclusive or chalked up to coincidence and other variables. Consumers have reported headaches, dizziness, digestive symptoms and mood swings as well as more serious health issues like Alzheimer's, birth defects, diabetes, hyperactivity and attention deficit disorders, Parkinson's disease, lupus, multiple sclerosis and seizures. However, studies on these effects have proved inconclusive as well. The most common additive used by the food industry are artificial flavorings with over 2000 different formulations currently in use. These chemicals are not required to be listed though some have been linked to allergic and behavioral reactions.

The refining process of wheat and other grains strips away the outer husk, leaving a refined starch which is easily broken down into sugar. This allows the starch to be absorbed into the bloodstream quickly which causes a rise in glucose levels and leads to obesity. Purchasing whole grains will ensure that the fibrous bran remains intact so that they are absorbed into the bloodstream more slowly. When the wheat germ and bran are removed during the milling process, so are the majority of key nutrients found in wheat. 50-93% of wheat's vitamin E, unsaturated fats, magnesium, zinc, chromium, manganese, calcium, phosphorous, potassium, iron, riboflavin, thiamin, niacin, and cobalt are lost during refining.

Chapter 5: Shopping Smart and Seasonal

Grocery shopping with clean eating in mind does not have to be daunting. With some knowledge and planning, you can become as well-versed and focused as a contestant on supermarket sweep! My number one advice when taking on the task of meal planning and grocery shopping for a clean diet is to think ahead. Sit down once a week and consider what you would like to eat. This book contains a few recipes to get you started. I also find that checking my local sale paper beforehand helps me to find a few deals and make the trip a bit easier on my bank account. As well as benefitting from sale papers and coupons, familiarize yourself with the harvest times of your favorite produce. Buying a mango when they are out of season will set you back almost double – sometimes more – than when they are in season. As well as the price, fruits and vegetables taste the best when they are not forced out of season. Ever eaten a peach so juicy and ripe that unintentionally utter slurping noises and somehow end up with your entire arm covered in sweet sticky nectar? Compare that to the misfortune of purchasing a peach during the fall. You bite into it only to experience a disappointing texture and less than desirable flavor. If the clean eating diet had a motto it would be, "Nature Knows Best." Gain some knowledge about crops that are grown in your area and their harvest times. Buying fresh, local, in season produce is a win-win. The items you purchase will undoubtedly be delicious and cost effective. You will also be supporting your local economy!

Now that you have planned your meals for the week and skimmed your sale paper, you are ready to take on the big box giants. Whenever possible, visit your local farmers market or you-pick field. Taking advantage of local produce, especially local honey, is a healthful and community-minded way to do your shopping. When you do venture into your supermarket, remember this major piece of advice: Shop the perimeter of the store. Most products lined up on the aisles are canned or boxed convenience foods that have been processed to oblivion in most cases so stick to the outer edges of the store in order to remove some guessing and label-reading from the equation.

Look for produce that is fresh and in season. Try not to just grab-and-go. Really stop and take a moment to examine the produce you are thinking of purchasing. You will need to employ all of your senses to help you pick a winner. Pick up the item that catches your eye and turn it over to check for brown spots and holes. The flesh should be firm but not rock hard and free of any dents or pits under the surface that may have occurred during shipping. Pay attention to the weight of the item in your hands. Especially with things like melons or oranges, heaviness can be the key to finding a juicy piece of fruit! Bring the item up and breathe it in. No, you do not have to make a spectacle of yourself by sniffing all of the produce in reach but you should detect a light sweet aroma. Strong or sour odor can suggest that what you are considering is approaching or already past its prime such as with melons and pineapple. Give squash and melons a little thump to determine ripeness and take that into consideration according to your meal plan. The produce planned for a meal toward the end of the week can afford to be a little less ripe than something you are cooking for dinner that night.

A number of the same rules for selecting fruit is applicable to vegetables, as well. The surface of the vegetable should be smooth, consistent, and evenly colored. An exception would be the squeeze test. Any give below the surface can indicate rotting and bruising. A firm texture is ideal. When evaluating leafy greens, you will want to observe a plumpness and regularity concerning the color of the leaves. You will want your greens to be smooth and snappy. However, some slight breakage and browning is a common side effect of the shipping process. If the majority of the leaves are smooth and unbroken, the few casualties of shipping can be looked over. Root vegetables such as carrots, turnips, potatoes, radishes, and onions should be firm and tough. If you notice any cracks and crevices around the base, it is an indicator that the vegetable has started to dry out.

Some produce will be shipped to stores with a wax coating in order to preserve freshness and prevent bruises during transit. Many fruits and vegetables produce a natural wax to help retain moisture which is usually washed off during processing and replaced with an artificial likeness. Keep this in mind when making your decision. An apple, for example, that is red and shiny but soft under the surface is probably not the best choice. If you buy produce that has been treated with wax, there is a method to removing it once you get home. Begin by getting rid of any stickers then gently scrub the surface under cold water a soft vegetable brush with to remove dirt and residue. Finally, plug your sink, fill it about halfway to the top with cold water, then add 3 or 4 cups of vinegar to make a solution depending on the volume of water you are using. The ideal ratio is 1 part vinegar to 3 parts water. Plunk your fruit into the solution and let it sit for about ten minutes.

A few tips for frugal folks: Shop in bulk. Some grocery chains display loose unpackaged foods such as nuts, olives, grains, and legumes. The cost that producers save on packaging is usually passed onto the consumer. Also, this way you can control the portion you buy to avoid spoiling. Bonus points for bringing reusable containers to store your goods! Avoid convenience foods. For example: vegetables that have already been chopped, bagged ready-to-eat salads, and shredded cabbage. These will more than likely cost much more than whole produce, create unnecessary waste due to the packaging, and more often than not are treated with even more preservatives to keep them fresh on the shelf for a longer period of time. Try to plan a few meals with alternative protein sources. Swapping an animal protein once a week for lentils, black beans, or tofu is going to make your wallet happy and reduce your fat intake without sacrificing on protein.

Chapter 6: Recipes for Breakfast

Cake Butter Chia Pudding with coconut whipped cream

Servings: 6

Ingredients

For the pudding

- 12 tbsp. chia seeds
- 2 cups unsweetened milk (You will need a little more when you are blending)
- 12 dates (Preferably medjool dates)
- ½ cup almond butter
- ½ cup oats (You could choose gluten free oats if you want)
- 2 tsp. Pure Vanilla Extract
- 3 tbsp. cacao nibs
- ½ tsp. almond extract

For the topping

- 2 cans coconut milk (leave it refrigerated overnight)
- 8 tsp. maple syrup
- 2 tsp. vanilla extract

Procedure

1. You will need to pit and cut the medjool dates.
2. Take a mixing bowl and add the chia seeds and the milk to the bowl. You will need to mix the ingredients well.
3. Now add the almond butter, dates and the oats. Mix the ingredients well and leave the bowl inside the refrigerator for an hour or two. You could also choose to leave it in the refrigerator overnight if you want.

4. Transfer the mixture in the bowl into a blender along with the cacao nibs.
5. Add the vanilla and the almond extract to the blender and a little bit of the milk. You will need to blend until you have a creamy and smooth mixture. Make sure that you add milk whenever you need to since you will need to ensure that the pudding is slightly thick. If you prefer a thicker pudding, you will need to add more milk and blend.
6. Taste the pudding and add more vanilla extract if you want to. You will also have to ensure that you balance the vanilla extract with the almond extract. If you want the pudding to be sweeter, you can add more dates to the blender and blend them in with the pudding. You will need to transfer the pudding into an airtight container and leave it in the refrigerator until it is cold. You will find that the mixture has begun to thicken inside the refrigerator.
7. While the mixture is chilling, you will need to make the topping. Open the can of the coconut milk and remove the solid white layer that is on top of the can. You have to ensure that you do not take any liquid along with the solid layer.
8. Add the solid layer to a metal bowl and beat the solid with four teaspoons of maple syrup and vanilla extract till the mixture has become fluffy. You can add more maple syrup if you desire. You will need to store this in the refrigerator.
9. Pull the pudding out and serve it in a bowl topped with the whipped cream and sprinkle some cacao nibs.

Oatmeal with Coconut, Amaranth and Maple Sautéed Apples

Servings: 4

Ingredients

- 2 cups rolled oats (preferably gluten free)

- 6 tbsp. amaranth seeds (If you prefer oats, you can add them instead of the amaranth)
- 2 cups coconut milk (you can take more if you need to. Make sure that you use light coconut milk as opposed to heavy)
- 2 cups almond milk
- A pinch of salt
- Ghee or Coconut oil
- 2 apples
- 2 tbsp. lemon juice
- 2 tbsp. water
- 4 tbsp. maple syrup
- 1 tsp. cinnamon (ground)
- Coconut flakes

Procedure

1. You will first need to core the apple and cut it into thin slices.
2. Take a medium sized skillet and place it on a medium flame. Add the oats, the coconut milk, almond milk and the amaranth to the skillet.
3. Bring the ingredients in the skillet to a boil while stirring them continuously. You will need to continue to simmer the ingredients till the oats have broken down. Make sure that there is a still a little pop left when it comes to the amaranth. You will need to continue to add milk in order to ensure that the ingredients do not burn.
4. While the ingredients are cooking, you will need to place a pan on a medium flame and add a little of the ghee or the coconut oil to the pan. Now add the apples to the pan and pour the lemon juice over the apples.
5. Add the water and maple syrup to the pan and mix the ingredients well. Add the cinnamon and give the apples a little flavor.
6. You will need to shake the pan well while ensuring that you do not move the apples around too much. Ensure that the

liquid moves around well. Cover the pan and leave the ingredients to cook on a medium flame. Make sure that you remove the pan off the heat when the apples have become soft.

7. Add one tablespoon of the apples to the skillet and cook the oats and the apples together. You will need to add the coconut flakes to the pan and cook the ingredients till the coconut flakes have turned golden brown. Remove the skillet from the heat immediately.

8. Transfer the oats to a bowl and serve with a topping of the apples and a few coconut flakes.

Banana Bread Breakfast Cookies

Servings: 30 cookies

Ingredients

- 4 bananas
- 2 cups oats (preferably gluten free)
- 2 tsp. vanilla extract
- 1 tbsp. chocolate chips
- 2 cups dried cranberries
- 2 cups walnuts
- 1 tbsp. Coconut flakes
- 2 tsp. Cacao nibs

Procedure

1. You will have to first cut and mash the bananas. Now, chop the walnuts. The walnuts do not have to be chopped too neatly. They can be chopped coarsely if you feel that the cookies will look better that way!

2. You will need to preheat the oven to 300 degrees Fahrenheit.

3. Add the oats to the blender and blend till the oats have the texture of flour! You will never have to use all – purpose

flour now. It is all right if the oats have not been ground finely.

4. Take a large bowl and add the mashed banana. Add the ground oats to the bowl and mix the ingredients till they have become smooth together. Now add the vanilla extract, chocolate chips, dried cranberries and the cacao nibs to the bowl. Mix the ingredients well together.
5. Take a baking tray and grease it well with coconut oil. You will need to scoop the mixture out of the bowl and press it firmly onto the baking tray. You will need to place the tray in the oven and bake the cookies for fifteen minutes. This is to ensure that the cookies have set.
6. Remove the tray from the oven and place it on the wire rack to cool.
7. Top the cookies with the coconut flakes and serve it warm with a glass of milk.

Breakfast Pasta

Servings: 2

Ingredients

- 2 cucumbers
- 2 zucchinis
- 2 tsp. lime juice
- 12 leaves of basil (preferably large)
- 2 cups berries (you can choose your favorite berries)
- 1 Apple
- 1 Kiwi fruit
- 2 tbsp. Poppy seeds
- 2 tbsp. Black sesame seeds
- 1 tbsp. shredded coconut

Procedure

1. You will first need to peel the cucumber and the zucchini using a vegetable peeler. You will need to keep the peeled skin aside. Make sure that the peeled skin is like a ribbon.
2. You will need to cut the basil leaves into ribbons too.
3. Dice the apple and the kiwi fruit and leave it in a bowl.
4. You will need to toss the ribbons of the cucumber and zucchini peels with the ribbons of the basil in a bowl. Add the lime juice to the bowl and toss the ribbons together one more time. Transfer these ribbons to a large bowl.
5. Add the remaining ingredients to the bowl and mix them well together. Make sure that you cut your berries before you add them to the bowl.
6. Transfer the pasta into two bowls and top the pasta with the shredded coconut and serve.

Sweet Potato Cakes

Servings: 4 – 6

Ingredients

- 2 pounds Sweet potatoes
- 4 tbsp. coconut oil (you could use any other healthy oil if you want to)
- ½ tsp. salt
- 4 eggs
- 2 cups coconut flour (Do not use All – purpose flour since that defies the rules of the diet)
- 1 tsp. coconut oil (for cooking)
- Salt and pepper to taste

Procedure

1. You will need to cube the sweet potatoes and add them to a large bowl of water and leave them to boil till they have become soft.

2. Now, remove the oil and begin to mash the potatoes using salt and oil to the potatoes. You will need to taste the potatoes in order to balance the flavor.
3. When the mashes potatoes are warm, you will need to add the eggs to the bowl and stir the eggs in with the potatoes.
4. Now add the coconut flour to the bowl and stir the ingredients together till you have obtained the consistency of the dough.
5. Now add remove the dough from the bowl and knead the dough gently with your hand. You have to be gentle since the dough is extremely soft. You will have to continue to add the flour to the bowl while kneading with your hand. Make sure that the ingredients do not stick together.
6. You will need to scoop the mixture and roll the dough out into a circle with the thickness of a quarter. You can use a bowl or a cup to cut the dough into circles.
7. Place the patties in a skillet that has been filled with the warm oil.
8. You will need to cook the patties in skillet on both sides till they have turned brown on both sides. They will burn quickly if you put the flame on high.
9. Serve the patties with maple syrup.

Skinny Omelet

Servings: 2

Ingredients

- 4 large eggs (make sure the eggs are organic)
- A pinch of salt
- 2 tbsp. Chives
- Two dollops of Pesto
- 1 tbsp. Goat Cheese
- 2 cups mixed salad greens

Procedure

1. You will need to chop the chives and place them in a bowl.
2. You will need to take a small bowl and crack the eggs in the bowl. Now beat the eggs using a fork. You will need to beat the eggs until the color is uniform. You will need to continue to beat the eggs well till there are no lumps.
3. Place a pan on a medium flame and add a little olive oil to the pan.
4. Now, pour half the egg mixture into the pan. You have to ensure that the egg mixture runs very well on the pan and that there are no patches of white and yellow on the pan.
5. Make sure that you spread the mixture out very thin onto the entire pan. You will need to sprinkle the chives onto the eggs and let them set. This will happen soon if your pan is hot.
6. You will need to run the spatula under the omelet and flip it onto the plate or on the countertop.
7. Now add the cheese to the top of the omelet. Add the salad greens and roll the omelet and serve it hot.
8. Do the same with the other half of the egg mixture and serve it hot.
9. You will need to add more salt to the omelet before you serve.

Porridge

Servings: 3 – 4

Ingredients

- 1 cup raw buckwheat groats
- 1 cup water
- 1 cup milk
- 2 tsp. cinnamon
- Vanilla

- 1 banana
- Toppings of your choice.

Procedure

You will need to take a bowl and add the ingredients to the bowl. Mix the ingredients well and add them to a blender. Leave the ingredients in the fridge overnight. Serve it warm with the toppings of your choice.

Chapter 7: Recipes for Mains

Black Bean Quinoa Salad

Servings: 8

Ingredients

For the Salad

- 2 cups quinoa
- 4 large navel oranges (cut into segments)
- 2 red bell peppers (diced)
- 2 cups jalapenos (seeded and diced)
- 2 cups black beans (canned, and water drained and rinsed)
- 1 cup corn kernels (canned and water drained)
- 4 tbsp. fresh cilantro leaves (chopped)
- 1 cup chopped red onion

For the orange vinaigrette

- 1 cup olive oil
- 1 cup apple cider vinegar
- 1 cup freshly squeezed orange juice
- 2 tbsp. Orange zest
- 1 tbsp. maple syrup

Procedure

1. Place a large saucepan on a medium flame and add two cups of the water to the pan. You will need to add the quinoa and cook it as per the instructions of the package. Set the pan aside.

2. You will now need to make the vinaigrette. You will need to add the ingredients for the vinaigrette in a small bowl and set that aside.
3. Take a large mixing bowl and add the oranges, quinoa, jalapeno, bell pepper onion, corn and cilantro. Mix the ingredients well together.
4. Pour the orange vinaigrette over the ingredients and toss the ingredients well together.
5. Serve it immediately.

Black Bean Soup

Servings: 6

Ingredients

For the Soup

- 8 tsp. Dried oregano leaves
- 2 tbsp. Salt (to taste)
- 6 cups dry black beans
- 4 tbsp. cumin
- 4 tbsp. oil
- 1 tsp. smoked paprika
- 24 cups Vegetable Broth
- 4 large bay leaves
- 4 onions
- 12 cloves garlic
- Cilantro (garnish)
- Sour Cream

For the Vegetable Stock

- 4 celery stalks
- 4 onions
- 4 carrots

- 20 florets Broccoli
- Sea Salt
- 16 cloves of garlic
- 4 cups green pepper
- 16 potatoes
- 1 lb. Beans
- Pepper
- 6 sprigs Thyme
- 6 sprigs Rosemary
- 4 sprigs Sage
- Fresh parsley

Procedure

For the Vegetable Stock

1. You will need to chop the vegetables coarsely or finely depending on your liking. They do not have to be chopped too finely.
2. You will need to take a large pot and add the vegetables to the pot.
3. You will next have to add the herbs to the pot along with the salt and pepper and mix the ingredients well together.
4. Add water to the pot while ensuring that three fourths of the pot is covered with water. This may be close to ten or fifteen cups of water.
5. Place this pot on a medium flame and let the water boil. You will need to reduce the flame and leave the ingredients in the water to simmer.
6. You will need to let the stock simmer for overran hour in order to obtain all the required nutrients.
7. You will need to continue to taste the stock repeatedly while it is stirring.
8. Once the stock has been on the flame for an hour, you will need to separate the stock from the vegetables. Set aside the required amount of stock for the soup.

For the Soup:

1. First soak the beans in water and then leave them in the sun to dry out.
2. Chop the onions and the garlic coarsely and set them aside.
3. Take a skillet and add a little oil to the pan. When the oil warms up, you will need to add the onions and the garlic to the pan and sauté the onions. The onions will need to become translucent and golden brown. You will then have to wait till the garlic has turned golden brown too.
4. Add the chipotle powder to the pan followed by the beans, the stock, bay leaves and the oregano to the pan.
5. Stir the ingredients well.
6. Cover the pan and turn the heat up to high. You will need to cook the ingredients well for tem minutes before you uncover the pan.
7. Now mix the ingredients well without the lid and let the ingredients in the pan warm up. Once the liquid has thickened, you will need to turn off the heat.
8. Remove the bay leaf from the pan and mash the beans. You will need to transfer the ingredients from the pan into a blender and make sure that the soup is smooth.
9. Now garnish the soup with the cilantro and the sour cream and serve it hot.

Creamy Tomato Basil Soup

Servings: 4

Ingredients

For the Soup
- 2 medium carrots, diced
- 2 stalks celery, diced
- 4 cloves garlic, minced

- 3 tbsp. butter
- 1 cup parmesan cheese, shredded
- 2 cans (14.5 ounce) chicken stock
- 2 medium onions, diced
- 4 tbsp. fresh basil
- 2 cups half and half
- 1 tsp. freshly ground black pepper
- 3 pounds tomatoes, cored, peeled, quartered
- 1 tbsp. tomato paste
- 1 tsp. salt or to taste

For the Chicken Stock

- 8 celery stalks
- 8 onions (halved and peeled)
- 4 cloves garlic 9halved)
- 12 Bay leaves
- 4 pounds chicken bones
- 8 carrots (peeled and cut)
- A bunch of parsley stems
- 8 sprigs thyme
- 2 tsp. Peppercorns (preferably black)

Procedure

For the Chicken Stock:

1. First preheat the oven to 300 degrees Fahrenheit and continue with the other tasks.
2. You will have to take a pan and roast the chicken bones on the pan and place it inside the oven. The bones have to be roasted well, which implies that they will need to be brown before you remove them off the pan.
3. Cut the vegetables coarsely. Now place a pan on the medium flame and add oil to the pan. When the oil has heated, you will need to add the vegetables to the pan and cook them well.

4. Wait till the onions have been cooked well. When the onions have turned golden brown and translucent, you will need to pull the vegetables off the pan.
5. Ensure that the other vegetables have also turned brown.
6. Now, add the vegetables to the pot and fill it with cold water. You will have to ensure that the vegetables have been covered well with the water. Remove the fat in the roasting pan and add the brown bits of the bones to the pot.
7. Place this pot on a medium flame and let the water boil. You will need to reduce the flame and leave the ingredients in the water to simmer.
8. You will need to let the stock simmer for overran hour in order to obtain all the required nutrients.
9. You will need to continue to taste the stock repeatedly while it is stirring.
10. Once the stock has been on the flame for an hour, you will need to separate the stock from the vegetables. Set aside the required amount of stock for the soup.

For the Soup:

1. Take a saucepan and place it on a medium flame. You will need to wait till the pan has warmed.
2. When the pan has warmed, add the butter to the pan and wait for it to melt. Once it has melted, you will need to add the onions, carrots and the celery to the pan.
3. You will need to cook the ingredients till the onions have turned translucent and are golden brown. Add the garlic to the pan now and cook till the fragrance has come.
4. Add the chicken stock to the pan along with the tomatoes, salt, pepper and the basil. You will need to mix the ingredients well.
5. Turn the heat up and cover the pan. Cook the ingredients on the high flame for ten minutes. Uncover the pan.

6. Now mix the ingredients well without the lid and let the ingredients in the pan warm up. Once the liquid has thickened, you will need to turn off the heat.

7. Remove the bay leaf from the pan and mash the beans. You will need to transfer the ingredients from the pan into a blender and make sure that the soup is smooth.

8. Add Parmesan and the half and half and serve hot.

Chicken, Chorizo and Kale Soup

Servings: 4

Ingredients

For the Soup
- 4 chicken thighs, skinless, boneless, diced
- 8 ounces pork chorizo, remove the casing
- 2 tbsp. olive oil
- 2 medium onions, finely chopped
- 2 cloves garlic, chopped, pressed
- 6 cups beef stock
- 2 bay leaves
- 15 ounce can diced tomatoes
- 15 ounce can chickpeas, drained, rinsed
- 4 medium Yukon gold potatoes, peeled, diced
- 5 ounces baby kale
- Salt to taste
- Pepper powder to taste

For the beef Stock
- 8 celery stalks
- 8 onions (halved and peeled)
- 4 cloves garlic 9halved)
- 12 Bay leaves
- 4 pounds beef bones

- 8 carrots (peeled and cut)
- A bunch of parsley stems
- 8 sprigs thyme
- 2 tsp. Peppercorns (preferably black)

Procedure

For the Beef Stock:

1. First preheat the oven to 300 degrees Fahrenheit and continue with the other tasks.
2. You will have to take a pan and roast the beef bones on the pan and place it inside the oven. The bones have to be roasted well, which implies that they will need to be brown before you remove them off the pan.
3. Cut the vegetables coarsely. Now place a pan on the medium flame and add oil to the pan. When the oil has heated, you will need to add the vegetables to the pan and cook them well.
4. Wait till the onions have been cooked well. When the onions have turned golden brown and translucent, you will need to pull the vegetables off the pan.
5. Ensure that the other vegetables have also turned brown.
6. Now, add the vegetables to the pot and fill it with cold water. You will have to ensure that the vegetables have been covered well with the water. Remove the fat in the roasting pan and add the brown bits of the bones to the pot.
7. Place this pot on a medium flame and let the water boil. You will need to reduce the flame and leave the ingredients in the water to simmer.
8. You will need to let the stock simmer for overran hour in order to obtain all the required nutrients.
9. You will need to continue to taste the stock repeatedly while it is stirring.

10. Once the stock has been on the flame for an hour, you will need to separate the stock from the vegetables. Set aside the required amount of stock for the soup.

For the soup

1. Place a pan on a medium flame and add the olive oil to the pan.
2. Add the onion to the pan and cook till the onions turn golden brown and have become translucent.
3. Now, add the chicken and the chorizo and cook till the chicken has turned brown on all sides.
4. Add the garlic to add a flavor to the chicken.
5. Now add the tomatoes, the stock, potatoes, kale and the bay leaves. Mix the ingredients well together.
6. Turn the heat up and cover the pan. Cook the ingredients on the high flame for ten minutes. Uncover the pan.
7. Now mix the ingredients well without the lid and let the ingredients in the pan warm up. Once the liquid has thickened, you will need to turn off the heat.
8. Remove the bay leaf from the pan and mash the beans. You will need to transfer the ingredients from the pan into a blender and make sure that the soup is smooth.
9. Add the chickpeas and serve it hot.

Easter Sunday Pot Roast

Servings: 4

Ingredients

For the sauce
- 1 packet instant gravy powder
- 1 packet instant ranch dip powder
- 2 cups beef broth
- 2 shallots, sliced

- 2 tbsp. Worcestershire sauce

For the roast

- 4 pounds beef rump roast
- 2 cups red potatoes, chopped
- 2 cups carrots, chopped
- 2 cups mushrooms, sliced
- 1 cup onions, sliced

For the beef Stock

- 8 celery stalks
- 8 onions (halved and peeled)
- 4 cloves garlic 9halved)
- 12 Bay leaves
- 4 pounds beef bones
- 8 carrots (peeled and cut)
- A bunch of parsley stems
- 8 sprigs thyme
- 2 tsp. Peppercorns (preferably black)

Procedure

For the Beef Stock:

11. First preheat the oven to 300 degrees Fahrenheit and continue with the other tasks.
12. You will have to take a pan and roast the beef bones on the pan and place it inside the oven. The bones have to be roasted well, which implies that they will need to be brown before you remove them off the pan.
13. Cut the vegetables coarsely. Now place a pan on the medium flame and add oil to the pan. When the oil has heated, you will need to add the vegetables to the pan and cook them well.
14. Wait till the onions have been cooked well. When the onions have turned golden brown and translucent, you will need to pull the vegetables off the pan.

15. Ensure that the other vegetables have also turned brown.
16. Now, add the vegetables to the pot and fill it with cold water. You will have to ensure that the vegetables have been covered well with the water. Remove the fat in the roasting pan and add the brown bits of the bones to the pot.
17. Place this pot on a medium flame and let the water boil. You will need to reduce the flame and leave the ingredients in the water to simmer.
18. You will need to let the stock simmer for overran hour in order to obtain all the required nutrients.
19. You will need to continue to taste the stock repeatedly while it is stirring.
20. Once the stock has been on the flame for an hour, you will need to separate the stock from the vegetables. Set aside the required amount of stock for the soup.

For the Roast:

1. You will need to place a skillet on a medium flame and add the ingredients of the sauce to the skillet.
2. You will need to mix all the ingredients well together and will need to add the vegetables and the roast to the pan. Mix the ingredients well and then cover the pan with a lid and cook the ingredients well together.
3. When the roast is cooked well, you will need to remove the pan off the flame and leave the pan aside.
4. Serve it hot after ten minutes.

Zucchini Boats

Serving: 4

Ingredients

- 4 cups zucchini
- ½ cup lentils

- ½ cup brown rice
- 6 cups water
- 2 onions
- 2 tomatoes
- 4 cloves garlic
- 1 red bell pepper
- 2 tsp. lemon juice
- 4 tbsp. olive oil
- 4 tbsp. pine nuts
- 4 tbsp. dried blueberries
- 4 tbsp. fresh mint
- 4 tbsp. fresh dill
- 4 tbsp. parsley
- ½ tsp. cinnamon (grounded)
- Salt and pepper

Procedure

1. You will need to chop all the vegetables and the herbs as well.
2. You will have to boil the rice and the lentils to make sure that they are soft but they will still be edible. You will need to drain the water out and set the lentils and the rice aside.
3. Cut the zucchinis lengthwise and make sure that there is enough room for all the filling.
4. Take a pan and add olive oil to the pan and place it on a medium flame. You will need to add the pine nuts and let them roast till they start changing in color.
5. Now add the onions to the pan and let them roast till they are golden brown and are translucent.
6. Add the bell pepper, the garlic, the tomatoes, black pepper and the cinnamon to the pan and cook the ingredients for another two minutes.
7. Now, add the rice and the lentils and cook the ingredients together for another few minutes.

8. You will need to add the greens and also the dried blueberries to the pan.
9. Fill the zucchini with the mix you have just made and put the zucchinis in the tray and bake them at 300 degrees Fahrenheit. You will need to cook the zucchinis for an hour. Now pull them out and add the lemon juice over them and serve them hot.

Chapter 8: Recipes for Desserts

Red Wine Poached Pears

Servings: 6

Ingredients

- 6 firm pears
- ½ bottle Red Wine (It is always good to select your favorite wine.)
- 1 Bay leaf
- 3 cloves (This is the spice)
- 1 tsp. Cinnamon
- 1 tsp. Ginger
- 1 ½ cups Maple Syrup
- 1 sprig Rosemary
- 1 sprigs Basil
- 1 sprig Sage

Procedure

1. First peel the pears and place them aside with their stems attached to the pear.
2. Take a skillet and add the wine into the skillet. Now add the cinnamon, maple syrup, ginger, cloves, and the bay leaf to the skillet. Mix the ingredients well to ensure that some of them have dissolved.
3. Now add the pears to the skillet and cover the skillet.
4. Place the skillet on a medium flame and leave it covered for ten minutes.
5. Pull the pears from the skillet and leave the pears aside. Leave the contents in the skillet to cook for a few seconds and let the wine thicken. Once the liquid has thickened, you will need to pour the liquid over the pears.

6. Garnish the pears with the herbs and serve them at room temperature.

Bread Pudding

Servings: 4

Ingredients

- 4 slices old bread, trim the crusts, cut into cubes
- 1 tbsp. butter
- ½ tsp. salt
- 1 cup golden raisins
- ½ tsp. ground cinnamon + extra to garnish
- ½ cup walnuts, chopped
- 2 cups warm milk
- 2 eggs, lightly beaten
- ½ cup packed, light brown sugar
- Zest of an orange, cut into very thin strips
- ½ tsp. vanilla extract
- 1 ½ cups water

Procedure

1. You will need a microwave dish and grease the dish with butter. Preheat the oven to 200 degrees Fahrenheit.
2. Take another bowl and add the bread, walnuts, orange zest and raisins together.
3. In another bowl, add the maple syrup, salt, cinnamon, milk, eggs and vanilla extract. You will need to pour this mixture into the bowl containing the bread. Cover the dish with a foil and transfer the bowl into the dish you have prepared with grease.
4. Now cook the mixture in the oven for ten minutes. When the time is up, you will need to pull the dish out and check whether or not the bread has cooked.

5. Sprinkle the dish with cinnamon powder and serve it hot!

Tapioca Pudding

Servings: 3

Ingredients

- 2 cups tapioca pearls, rinsed, drained
- 5 cups whole milk
- 2 cups maple syrup
- 2 tsp. vanilla extract
- 2 cups water

Method:

1. Preheat the oven to 400 degrees Fahrenheit.
2. You will need to prepare a dish and line it with grease.
3. Take a bowl and add the ingredients to the bowl. Mix them well to ensure that there is a balance of flavor. If you want the dish to be sweeter, you will need to add more maple syrup.
4. Transfer this mixture into the prepared bowl and place the bowl in the oven.
5. When the cooking is done, you will need to remove the bowl from the oven and stir the contents violently.
6. Transfer the contents into serving bowls and cover them with wraps to let them set.
7. Serve them cold.

Stuffed Peaches

Servings: 12

Ingredients

- 8 cups water

- 32 Gingersnap or Amaretto Cookies
- 8 tbsp. Almonds
- 8 tbsp. Butter
- 4 tsp. lemon zest
- 12 firm peaches

Procedure

1. Preheat the oven to 300 degrees Fahrenheit.
2. First crumble the cookies and chop all the almonds. They can be chopped coarsely if you prefer.
3. Cut the peaches into halves and make sure that you pit them.
4. Now add two cups of water to a large bowl and leave it in the refrigerator.
5. Take another bowl and add the crumbs of the cookies, the lemon zest and the almonds to the bowl and mix them well together.
6. Stuff the peaches with this mixture and transfer the peaches into the baking tray. Leave the tray in the bowl containing the water and cook for ten minutes.
7. You will now have to remove the peaches and serve them warm with a scoop of chocolate or vanilla ice cream.

Chapter 9: Sample Shopping List and Meal Plans

This chapter contains a few sample meal plans that you can use. If you are able to stick to this plan, you can motivate yourself to do better and keep yourself fit and strong.

Day 1:

Breakfast: Breakfast Pasta

Lunch: Easter Sunday pot Roast + Black bean Soup

Snack: Tapioca Pudding

Dinner: Zucchini Boats + Black Bean Quinoa Salad

Day 2:

Breakfast: Sweet Potato Cakes

Lunch: Chorizo, Chicken and Kale Soup + Skinny Omelet

Snack: Stuffed Peaches

Dinner: Creamy tomato Basil Soup + Red Wine Poached Pears

Day 3:

Breakfast: Banana Bread Breakfast Cookies

Lunch: Porridge + Black Bean Soup

Snack: Cake Butter Chia Pudding

Dinner: Zucchini Boats + Black Bean Quinoa Salad

Week 1 –

Proteins and Dairy

- 2 oz. Grated Parmesan Cheese

- 9 oz. Ricotta Cheese
- 5 ½ oz. Cottage Cheese
- 2 Dozen Large Eggs
- 21 oz. Plain Whole-Milk Greek Yogurt
- 4 oz. Lean Ground Bison
- 3 oz. Lean Beef Tenderloin
- 8 oz. Lean Ground Turkey
- 2 oz. Thinly Sliced Deli Turkey (No Added Nitrates or Nitrites)
- 1 pkg. Lean Uncured Turkey Bacon (No Added Nitrates Nitrites)
- 14 oz. Boneless, Skinless Chicken Breasts
- 1 lb. Boneless, Skinless Chicken Tenders (Freeze Half for Week 2)
- 4 oz. Smoked Wild Alaskan Salmon
- 4 oz. Can of Wild Tuna (Packed in Water)

Veggies and Fruits

- 2 Apples
- 4 Bananas (Freeze 1)
- 2 Lemons
- 1 Lime
- 1 Orange
- 1 Grapefruit
- 16 oz. Fresh Strawberries
- 12 oz. Fresh Blueberries
- 2 Pears
- 2 Avocados
- 6 ½ oz. Carrots (3 Medium)
- 2 Stalks Celery
- 2 Red Bell Peppers
- 2 Cucumbers (1 English)
- 2 Large Zucchini

- 1 pt. Grape Tomatoes
- 1 Small Head of Broccoli
- 5 oz. Mushrooms
- 1 Large Yellow Onion
- 1 Shallot
- 1 Bunch of Green Onion
- 1 Head of Garlic
- 5 ½ oz. Baby Spinach
- 1 Head Bibb or Butter Lettuce
- 1 Large Bunch of Cilantro
- 1 Bunch of Fresh Rosemary
- 2 Sweet Potatoes
- 1 Small Yukon Gold Potato
- 2 Medjool Dates

Whole Grains

- 1 Loaf sprouted whole-grain bread (Try Food for Life Ezekiel 4:9 Flax Sprouted Whole Grain Bread)
- 1 pkg. 8-Inch Sprouted Grain Tortillas
- 1 Container Old-Fashioned Rolled Oats
- 1 Bag Brown Rice
- 1 Bag Quinoa (Try NOW Foods Living Now Certified Organic Whole Grain Quinoa)

Nuts, Seeds, and Oils

- 1 Jar Ghee (Clarified Butter) or 1 Stick Organic Unsalted Butter
- 1 Bottle Extra Virgin Olive Oil
- 1 Bottle Olive Oil
- 1 Jar Unrefined Coconut Oil
- 1 Jar Raw Almond Butter
- 2 oz. Raw Unsalted Chopped Walnuts
- 2 oz. Unsalted Pine Nuts
- 1 oz. Raw Unsalted Almonds

- 1 Bag Ground Flaxseed
- 1 Bag Chia Seeds (Try Nutiva Organic Chia Seeds)
- 1 Bag Hemp Hearts (Raw Shelled Hemp Seeds)

Extras

- 32 oz. Carton Unsweetened Vanilla Almond Milk
- 12 oz. Low-Sodium Vegetable Broth
- 15 oz. BPA-Free Can of Unsalted Black Beans
- 16 oz. Bag Frozen Shelled Edamame
- 1 Bag Red Lentils
- 1 Bag Almond Flour
- 1 pkg. Nori (Seaweed Sheets)
- 1 Jar All-Natural Mango Salsa
- 1 Jar All-Natural Salsa
- 1 ½ oz. Dried Unsweetened Cranberries
- 8 oz. Container of Hummus
- 1 Jar Dijon Mustard
- 1 Jar Raw Honey
- 1 Bottle Rice Vinegar
- 1 Bottle Ground Cinnamon
- 1 Bottle Ground Oregano
- 1 Bottle Ground Cumin
- 1 Bottle Smoked Paprika
- 1 Jar Wasabi Paste
- 1 Bottle Ground Black Pepper
- 1 Bottle Sea Salt
- 1 Box Baking Powder
- 1 Bottle Pure Vanilla Extract

Week 2-

Proteins and Dairy

- 22 oz. Plain Whole-Milk Greek Yogurt

- 8 oz. Medium Shrimp
- 9 oz. Thinly Sliced Deli Turkey (No Added Nitrates or Nitrites)
- 8 oz. Wild Halibut Fillet
- 4 oz. Wild Smoked Alaskan Salmon
- 8 oz. Extra-Firm Organic Tofu

Veggies and Fruits

- 2 Apples
- 2 Bananas
- 15 oz. Fresh Strawberries (Slice and Freeze 9 oz.)
- 13 oz. Blueberries
- 1 Pear
- 1 Orange
- 1 Lime
- 1 Cucumber
- 1 Papaya
- 1 Pineapple
- 2 Avocados
- 4 oz. Snap Peas
- 1 Red Bell Pepper
- 1 Large Zucchini
- 1 Medium Yellow Onion
- 1 Bunch Green Onions
- 1 Sweet Potato
- 2 Small Purple Potatoes
- 4 Portobello Mushroom Caps
- 4 oz. Shiitake Mushrooms
- 1 Large Bunch Fresh Cilantro
- 6 oz. Field Greens
- 1 Head Bok Choy

Whole Grains

- 1 Bag Oat Flour

Nuts, Seeds, and Oils

- 1 Bottle Toasted Sesame Oil
- 1 Bottle Grapeseed Oil

Extras

- 1 Jar Low-Sugar Marinara Sauce
- 4 oz. Bag Shirataki Noodles
- 1 Bottle Wheat-Free Low Sodium Tamari Sauce
- 1 Container Baking Soda
- 1 Bottle Sriracha Sauce
- 1 Bottle Apple Cider Vinegar
- 1 Bag Coconut Sugar
- 15 oz. BPA-Free Can Unsalted Black Beans
- 5 oz. BPA-Free Can Water Chestnuts
- 1 Jar Water-Packed Roasted Red Peppers
- 1 Jar or Can Chipotle Chiles in Adobo Sauce
- 1 Bottle Ground Chile Powder
- 1 Bottle Cracked Black Pepper
- 1 Bag Arrowroot
- 8 oz. Container Hummus

Week 1

Monday:

Breakfast

- 1 slice of sprouted-grain bread (toasted) with ¼ avocado (mashed)
- ¼ cup of spinach and 1 soft boiled egg
- ½ grapefruit

Snack

- 1 pear
- 8 almonds

Lunch

- 1 serving of nori-wrapped salmon hand rolls*
- ½ cup cooked brown rice
- ½ cup steamed edamame

Snack

- Sonoma salad
  (6 oz. cooked and diced chicken breast, 2 stalks chopped celery, ½ chopped apple, 1 tbsp. hemp seeds, 1 tbsp. chopped almonds. For the dressing: ½ cup Greek yogurt and 2 tbsp. lemon juice. 1 sprouted whole grain tortilla)

Dinner

- Steak kabobs*

  Total Daily Nutrition
  Calories: 1,627
  Fat: 71g
  Saturated fats: 15g
  Carbs: 152g
  Fiber: 30g
  Sugars: 48g
  Protein: 101g
  Sodium: 1,075mg
  Cholesterol: 434mg

Tuesday:

Breakfast

- Yogurt berry bowl
  (Mix ¾ cup Greek yogurt, 1 cup sliced strawberries, 2 tbsp. chopped walnuts and 1 tbsp. chia seeds)

Snack

- 1 slice sprouted-grain bread, toasted, with 1/3 cup cottage cheese and ¼ cup mango salsa

Lunch

- 1 serving nori-wrapped salmon hand rolls
- ¾ cup cooked brown rice
- ½ cup edamame, steamed

Snack

- 1 banana, sliced, dip in 1 tbsp. ground flaxseed

Dinner

- Turkey taco lettuce wraps
(Mix 4 oz. cooked ground turkey, ½ cup cooked brown rice, ¼ cup salsa, ¼ cup black beans, ¼ avocado, cubed, 2 tbsp. chopped green onion and 2 tbsp. chopped red pepper; serve in Bibb lettuce leaves)

Total Daily Nutrition
Calories: 1,546
Fat: 65g
Saturated fat: 18g
Carbs: 170g
Fiber: 33g
Sugars: 56g
Protein: 84g
Sodium: 1,988mg
Cholesterol: 357mg

Wednesday:

Breakfast

- 1 serving protein pancakes with berry coulis*
- 2 strips turkey bacon; cooked
- 1 egg, hard-boiled
- ½ grapefruit

Snack

- ½ cucumber, sliced
- 1 carrot, sliced
- 2 tbsps. hummus
- 2 oz. deli turkey

Lunch

- Tuna salad
  (Mix 1 can tuna with 1 tbsp. Dijon mustard, 1 tbsp. Greek yogurt and 1 green onion, chopped; serve over 1 cup baby spinach, ¼ cup cooked quinoa, ½ cup chopped cucumber and 1 carrot, chopped.)

Snack

- 1 banana, sliced; dip in 1 tbsp. ground flaxseed
- ½ apple, sliced, with 2 tbsps. almond butter
- 1/3 cup cottage cheese

Dinner:

- Smoky lentils & quinoa*

Total Daily Nutrition
Calories: 1,488
Fat: 52g
Saturated fat: 8g
Carbs: 158g

Fiber: 37g
Sugars: 54g
Protein: 99g
Sodium: 1,699mg
Cholesterol: 446m

Thursday:

Breakfast

- 1 serving veggie-filled egg muffins*
- 1 apple, sliced; sautéed in 1 tsp. coconut oil and sprinkled with cinnamon

Snack

- 1 cup strawberries
- 8 almonds

Lunch

- Smoky lentils and quinoa (leftovers), reheated

Snack

- Banana nut butter shake
  (Blend 1 cup almond milk, ½ frozen banana, 1 tbsp. almond butter, 1 tbsp. hemp seeds, and 1 Medjool date with ice)

Dinner

- 1 serving zoodles with cilantro pesto & grilled chicken* (save leftovers)

Total Daily Nutrition
Calories: 1,592
Fat: 78g
Saturated fat: 20g

Carbs: 161g
Fiber: 40g
Sugars: 65g
Protein: 74g
Sodium: 1,177mg
Cholesterol: 258mg

Friday:

Breakfast

- Yogurt berry bowl
  (Mix ¾ cup Greek yogurt, 1 cup blueberries, 2 tbsps. chopped almonds, and 1 tbsp. chia seeds.)

Snack

- ½ cucumber, sliced,
- 1 carrot, sliced
- 2 tbsps. Hummus

Lunch

- 1 serving veggie-filled egg muffins (leftovers)
- ½ cup cooked quinoa mixed with 2 tbsps. dried cranberries, 2 tbsps. pine nuts and 1 tbsp. rice vinegar

Snack

- Sonoma salad (leftovers)
- 1 sprouted-grain tortilla

Dinner

- Rosemary chicken
  (Sauté 1 clove minced garlic, 1 chopped Yukon Gold potato, and ¼ cup chopped yellow onion in 1 tsp ghee; set aside on a

plate. Sauté 4 oz. chopped chicken breast, and 1 tbsp. rosemary in 1 tsp ghee. When chicken is done, return vegetables to pan and toss.)

Total Daily Nutrition
Calories: 1,771
Fat: 77g
Saturated fat: 25g
Carbs: 156g
Fiber: 30g
Sugars: 42g
Protein: 124g
Sodium: 1,079mg
Cholesterol: 244mg

Saturday:

Breakfast

- 1 serving protein pancakes with berry coulis (leftovers) reheated
- 2 strips turkey bacon, cooked

Snack

- Yogurt berry bowl
(Mix ¾ cup Greek yogurt, 1 cup blueberries, 1 tbsp. chia seeds and 1 tsp honey.)

Lunch

- Turkey taco lettuce wraps
(Mix 4 oz. cooked ground turkey, ½ cup cooked brown rice, ¼ cup salsa, ¼ cup black beans, ¼ avocado, cubed, 2 tbsps. chopped green onion and 2 tbsps. chopped red bell pepper; serve in Bibb lettuce leaves)

Snack

- Banana nut butter shake
  (Blend 1 cup almond milk, ½ frozen banana, 1 tbsp. almond butter, 1 tbsp. hemp seeds and 1 Medjool date with ice)

Dinner

- 1 serving zoodles with cilantro and grilled chicken (leftovers) reheated

  Total Daily Nutrition
  Calories: 1,559
  Fat: 69g
  Saturated fat: 16g
  Carbs: 146g
  Fiber: 31g
  Sugars: 70g
  Protein: 106g
  Sodium: 1,787mg
  Cholesterol: 321mg

Sunday:

Breakfast

- 1 slice sprouted-grain bread, toasted, with ¼ avocado, mashed
- ¼ cup spinach and 1 egg, soft-boiled
- ½ cup strawberries

Snack

- 1 pear sprinkled with 1 tbsp. hemp seeds
- 1 tbsp. walnuts

Lunch

- Baja salad
  (Mix 4 oz. grilled and chopped chicken breast, ½ cup cooked quinoa, ½ cup black beans, 6 sliced grape tomatoes, 1 tbsp. chopped green onion, 1 tbsp. cilantro leaves, juice of 1 lime and 1/8 tsp cumin.)

Snack

- 1 slice sprouted-grain bread, toasted
- ½ tbsp. almond butter
- ½ banana, sliced

Dinner

- 4 oz. ground bison; form into a patty and grilled
- 1½ cups broccoli florets, sautéed in 1 tsp ghee
- 1 sweet potato, baked

Total Daily Nutrition
Calories: 1,319
Fat: 37g
Saturated fat: 8g
Carbs: 152g
Fiber: 30g
Sugars: 36g
Protein: 95g
Sodium: 944mg
Cholesterol: 386mg

* Nori-Wrapped Salmon Hand Rolls with Wasabi Aioli

In a large bowl, whisk together 1 large egg yolk, 1 tsp. Dijon and 1 tsp. wasabi paste. Slowly drizzle in EVOO while whisking vigorously until mixture thickens. Mix in 1 tsp. fresh lemon juice. Set aside.

Lay 2 sheets of nori cut in half on a flat surface. Lay 1 oz. salmon along one side of each sheet, toward one of the corners. Divide ½ English cucumber cut into matchsticks, ½ sliced avocado and 2 tbsp. chopped fresh cilantro among nori, layering over salmon. Starting from the corner with filling, roll into a cone shape. (You may need a few drops of water to seal.) Serve with aioli.

Tip: refrigerate 1 serving of rolls and sauce; alternatively, you can save half the ingredients for the rolls and wrap them freshly the next day.

*Steak Kabobs

Make skewers from 3 oz. beef, cut into chunks, 4 grape tomatoes, 1 zucchini, cut into rounds. Brush with 1 tsp. EVOO and sprinkle with salt and pepper. Grill 1 baked sweet potato.

*Protein Pancakes with Berry Coulis

Place ½ cup old-fashioned oats in a blender; pulse until a powder forms. Add 2 large eggs, 1/3 cup of ricotta cheese, 1 tbsp. ground flaxseed, 2 tsp. baking powder, 1 tsp. pure vanilla extract, ¼ tsp ground cinnamon and 1 tsp. raw honey. Blend until smooth. Transfer batter to a bowl and clean out blender.

Heat an electric griddle or cast-iron skillet to 325°F and coat surface with oil. Add 1 heaping tbsp. batter per pancake and cook until bubbles form on the surface of batter, about 2 minutes. Flip and cook until golden, 2 minutes more.

In clean blender, combine ¼ cup blueberries, ¼ cup chopped strawberries and 2 tbsps. fresh squeezed orange juice. Process until roughly blended. Serve coulis over pancakes.

*Smoky Lentils and Quinoa

Cook ½ cup of chopped yellow onion, 1 minced garlic clove, 1 chopped red bell pepper, ½ cup red lentils, ½ cup rinsed quinoa and ½ tsp. smoked paprika in 1 ½ cups of vegetable stock. Bring to boil, and then reduce to simmer. Cover and cook about 15 minutes. (eat half and save the leftovers)

*Veggie-Filled Egg Muffins

Preheat oven to 350°F. Coat 8 cups of a regular muffin tin with olive oil cooking spray. Combine 8 tbsps. almond flour with 8 tsps. coconut oil. Divide evenly among the bottoms of the prepared muffin cups and flatten down with your fingers. Bake for 10 minutes, or until golden brown.

Coat a medium-sized nonstick skillet with olive oil cooking spray and turn on medium-high. Add in 2 cups sliced mushrooms and ¼ cup chopped yellow onion then cook until soft, about 4 minutes. Lastly, add in the 2 cups baby spinach and finish cooking vegetables until spinach is wilted. Set aside the cooked vegetables in a separate bowl to cool for about 5 minutes.

In a large bowl, whisk 4 large eggs, 4 egg whites, 1/4 cup grated parmesan cheese and black pepper. Add vegetables to the egg and cheese mixture. Divide finished mixture among the muffin cups about 3/4 full and add the remaining 4 tsp parmesan on top. Bake about 17 minutes until light golden brown and puffed.

*Zoodles with Cilantro Pesto and Grilled Chicken

For this recipe, you will need a spiral maker (Directions vary by brand so be sure to read over before beginning). Set zucchini in the spiral maker and turn the crank to produce your "zoodles" in long strands to mimic spaghetti noodles. Spread zoodles out onto a double layer of paper towels then gently squeeze with more paper towels to remove any excess moisture. Add a pinch of salt over the top to draw out the last bit of moisture and set aside for 30 to 45 minutes. Work in small batches and gently squeeze out whatever moisture remains.

In your food processor, pulse 2 cups of cilantro, 2 tbsps. chopped unsalted walnuts, 2 tbsps. chopped shallot, 1 ½ tbsps. Parmesan cheese, zest and juice of half of a lemon, 2 small cloves of minced garlic and ½ tsp. dried oregano. Add in 1 tbsp. olive oil while machine is running. Set aside.

Place chicken breast tenders between 2 sheets of wax paper or cling wrap. Pound them out to about 1-inch in thickness. In a large skillet heated to medium-high, add ½ tsp oil. After seasoning chicken with pepper, cook for 4 to 6 minutes on each side. Set the chicken aside and let rest for 5 minutes before slicing.

Coat the skilled with olive oil cooking spray and heat to med-high. Cook zoodles for 2 to 3 minutes, until they soften slightly. Remove the zoodles from pan and toss with the pesto that was set aside. Plate the pesto zoodles and top with sliced chicken.

Week 2

Monday:

Breakfast

- 1 serving sweet potato hash with sunny side up eggs* (save leftovers)

Snack

- 1 serving mini blueberry muffins* (save leftovers)

Lunch

- 1 serving black bean patty salad* (save leftovers)

Snack

- 1 serving purple potato egg salad* (save leftovers)

Dinner

- 1 serving Polynesian stir-fry* (save leftovers)

Total Daily Nutrition
Calories: 1,732
Fat: 71.5g
Saturated fat: 15g
Carbs: 205g
Fiber: 39g
Sugars: 61g
Protein: 71.5g
Sodium: 2,074mg
Cholesterol: 511mg

Tuesday

Breakfast

- Yogurt berry bowl

  (Mix ¾ cup Greek yogurt, 1 cup sliced strawberries, 1 tbsp. chopped walnuts and 1 tbsp. chia seeds.)

Snack

- Strawberry smoothie

(Blend ¾ cup frozen strawberries, ¼ cup Greek yogurt, ¼ cup almond milk, 1 tbsp. chia seeds, 1½ tsp ground flaxseed and 1 tsp honey with ice)

Lunch

- Smoked salmon bowl

(Top ½ cup cooked quinoa with ½ cup edamame, steamed, 2 oz. smoked salmon,   2 tbsps. each chopped cucumber and avocado, 1 tbsp. chopped cilantro; drizzle   with ½ tsp each tamari and rice vinegar)

Snack

- Turkey wrap

(1 tortilla, add 2 tbsps. hummus, 3 oz. deli turkey, 1/8 avocado, sliced, and 2   tbsps. cilantro)

Dinner

- Papaya shrimp

(Sauté ½ cup chopped yellow onion, 2 cloves minced garlic, 8 oz. shrimp and ½ papaya, peeled and chopped, in 2 tsp ghee. Eat half over 2 oz. shirataki noodles.   Save leftovers)

Total Daily Nutrition
Calories: 1,448
Fat: 59g
Saturated fat: 13g
Carbs: 129g
Fiber: 35g
Sugars: 45g
Protein: 112g
Sodium: 1,578mg
Cholesterol: 273mg

Wednesday

Breakfast

- 1 serving sweet potato hash with sunny side up eggs (leftovers) reheat

Snack

- 1 serving mini blueberry muffins (leftovers)

Lunch

- 1 serving black bean patty salad (leftovers)

Snack

- 1 serving purple potato egg salad (leftovers)

Dinner

- 1 serving Polynesian stir-fry (leftovers) reheat

Total Daily Nutrition
Calories: 1,732
Fat: 71.5g
Saturated fat: 15g
Carbs: 205g
Fiber: 39g
Sugars: 61g
Protein: 71.5g
Sodium: 2,074mg
Cholesterol: 511mg

Thursday

Breakfast

- 1 serving veggie-filled egg muffins (leftovers) reheat

- 1 apple, sliced; sauté in 1 tsp coconut oil and sprinkle with cinnamon

Snack

- Turkey wrap

(1 tortilla, add 2 tbsps. hummus, 3 oz. deli turkey, 1/8 avocado, sliced, and 2   tbsps. cilantro)

Lunch

- Portobello mushroom pizzas*

- 1/3 cup cooked quinoa mixed with 2 tbsps. dried cranberries, 1 tbsp. pine nuts and 1 tbsp. rice vinegar

Snack

- 1 slice sprouted-grain bread, toasted

- 1 tbsp. almond butter

- ¼ papaya, sliced

Dinner

- Papaya Shrimp (reheat leftovers) over 2 oz. shirataki noodles

Total Daily Nutrition
Calories: 1,618
Fat: 77g
Saturated fat: 31g
Carbs: 150g
Fiber: 30g

Sugars: 55g
Protein: 95g
Sodium: 1,977mg
Cholesterol: 448mg

Friday

Breakfast

- 1 serving protein pancakes with berry coulis (leftovers) thawed and reheated

- 2 strips turkey bacon, cooked

- 1 banana

Snack

- Yogurt berry bowl

(Mix ½ cup Greek yogurt, 1 cup blueberries, 1 tbsp. chia seeds and 1 tbsp. ground   flaxseed.)

Lunch

- Smoked salmon bowl

(Top ½ cup cooked quinoa with ½ cup steamed edamame, 2 oz. smoked salmon, 2 tbsps. each chopped cucumber and avocado, 1 tbsp. chopped cilantro; drizzle   with ½ tsp each tamari and rice vinegar.)

Snack

- ¼ papaya, sliced

- 1 tbsp. chopped walnuts

Dinner

- 1 serving zoodles with cilantro pesto and grilled chicken (leftovers)

Total Daily Nutrition
Calories: 1,453
Fat: 63g
Saturated fat: 13g
Carbs: 132g
Fiber: 31g
Sugars: 60g
Protein: 103g
Sodium: 1,379mg
Cholesterol: 299mg

Saturday

Breakfast

- 1 serving veggie-filled egg muffins (leftovers) thawed and reheated

- 1 apple, sliced; sauté in 1 tsp coconut oil and sprinkle with cinnamon

Snack

- ½ banana, sliced; dip in 1 tbsp. almond butter and 1 tbsp. ground flaxseed

Lunch

- 1 serving zoodles with cilantro pesto & grilled chicken (leftovers) reheated

Snack

- Yogurt berry bowl

Dinner

- Halibut with vegetables

(In a large piece of foil, place 8 oz. halibut fillet, 2 cups shredded bok choy, 6 sliced shiitake mushrooms, 2 tbsps. fresh cilantro, 1 tbsp. rice vinegar and 1 tbsp. tamari. Wrap and fold foil to enclose food then bake packet at 350°F for 15 minutes. Eat half with ¾ cup cooked brown rice and save leftovers.)

Total Daily Nutrition
Calories: 1,475
Fat: 56g
Saturated fat: 14g
Carbs: 158g
Fiber: 35g
Sugars: 69g
Protein: 97g
Sodium: 1,504mg
Cholesterol: 344mg

Sunday

Breakfast

- 1 serving protein pancakes with berry coulis (leftovers) thawed and reheated

- 2 strips turkey bacon, cooked

- 1 pear

Snack

- Quinoa turkey snack

(Mix ½ cup cooked quinoa with 2 tbsps. dried cranberries, 1 tbsp. pine nuts, 1   tbsp. rice vinegar and 3 oz. deli turkey, chopped)

Lunch

- Halibut with vegetables (leftovers), reheated, with ¾ cup cooked brown rice

Snack

- Strawberry smoothie

(Blend ¾ cup frozen strawberries, ¼ cup Greek yogurt, ¼ cup almond milk, 1 tbsp. chia seeds, 1½ tsp ground flaxseed and 1 tsp. honey with ice)

Dinner

- Portobello Mushroom Pizzas

Total Daily Nutrition
Calories: 1,506
Fat: 53g
Saturated fat: 18g
Carbs: 165g
Fiber: 33g
Sugars: 54g
Protein: 103g
Sodium: 2,097mg
Cholesterol: 290 mg

*Sweet Potato Hash with Sunny Side Up Eggs

Mist a large nonstick skillet with cooking spray and heat on medium-high. To skillet, add 1/3 cup chopped yellow onion, 2 1-oz. slices of all-natural turkey bacon, chopped and sauté for 4 minutes until onion is translucent. Add 1 shredded sweet potato, salt and pepper and sauté about 8 minutes. Add the cilantro before plating the hash.

Reduce heat to medium and mist same skillet with olive oil cooking spray. Cook the 2 large eggs on opposite sides of the prepared skillet and cook until set. Add 1 egg over the top of each serving of hash.

*Mini Blueberry Muffins

Preheat oven to 350°F. Mist a mini muffin tin with cooking spray or line with paper cups.

In a large mixing bowl, whisk together 1 cup of almond flour and ¼ tsp. of baking soda. In another medium bowl, whisk together 2 large eggs, 2 tbsps. raw honey, ½ tsp. pure vanilla extract, ½ tsp. apple cider vinegar, ¾ tsp. cinnamon and a pinch of sea salt. Pour into flour mixture and mix until combined. Fold in ½ cup frozen wild blueberries.

Place about 1 tbsp. of batter in each of 16 muffin cups. Bake for 15 minutes or until golden.

*Black Bean Patty Salad

To a food processor, add ½ cup cooked quinoa, ¼ cup oat flour, 2/3 cup unrinsed black beans, ½ cup roasted red pepper, ½ cup chopped yellow onion, ¼ chopped fresh cilantro, 1 clove of garlic, 1 tsp. chile powder, zest and juice of ½ lime, 1 tsp. cumin, ½ tsp. smoked paprika and 1/4 tsp. sea salt. Pulse until combined into a patty texture. Transfer to a mixing bowl and fold in remaining black beans.

To a large pan on medium-high, add oil. Form 5 patties and flatten slightly. Cook patties for 4 minutes on each side, until golden. Divide field greens mix, ½ cup salsa and 12 halved grape tomatoes between 2 bowls. Top each with 1 black bean patty and half of a sliced avocado on each patty.

Whisk together ½ cup Greek yogurt, zest and juice of ½ lime, ½ chipotle pepper, 1 tbsp. adobo sauce and 1/8 tsp salt. Divide sauce over top of each salad.

*Purple Potato Egg Salad

Place 2 chopped purple potatoes in a deep saucepan and top with cold water. Bring cold water up to a boil, reduce to simmer and cook about 8 minutes or until fork tender. Drain and then set potatoes aside in a large bowl.

To another saucepan, add 2 large eggs and cover with cold water then bring to a boil on med-high. Set timer for 10 minutes; drain the water and let sit for 1 additional minute. Fill a large bowl with cold water and a tbsp. of baking soda to peel. Chop the eggs then add them to the bowl with the potatoes.

To a small skillet over medium heat, add 2 1-oz slices of turkey bacon and cook about 2-4 minutes per side depending on preference. Chop the cooked turkey bacon and one green onion then add to the potatoes and boiled eggs.

For the dressing, whisk together 2 tbsps. apple cider vinegar, 2 tbsps. Dijon mustard, 1 tbsp. olive oil, and black pepper to taste. Pour prepared dressing over the egg-potato mixture and stir to coat.

*Polynesian Stir-Fry

To a small saucepan, add ½ cup brown rice and 1 cup water. Bring to boil then cover and reduce to simmer until tender, about 35 to 40 minutes.

For the sauce, whisk together 2 tbsp. apple cider vinegar, 1 tbsp. reduced sodium tamari, 3 tbsps. fresh squeezed orange juice, 1 tbsp. coconut sugar and sriracha to taste.

In a large nonstick skillet or wok on high, add 1 tsp. grape seed oil. To the oil, add 1 cup snap peas, 1 cup diced red bell pepper, ¾ cup fresh pineapple, 4 chopped green onions and 5 oz. can of water chestnuts. Stir-fry for 4 minutes then transfer to a plate.

In the same pan, add remaining 1 tsp grape seed oil. Add 8 oz. extra-firm tofu and brown for 2 minutes on each side. Return sauce and vegetables to pan. When bubbles start to form, add mixture of 1 tsp. each water and arrowroot. Let simmer for about 15 seconds, and then stir to coat. Drizzle 1 tsp. toasted sesame oil on top. Serve over rice.

*Portobello Mushroom Pizzas

Remove gills from 2 Portobello mushroom caps. Fill each cap with 2 tbsp. marinara sauce and ¼ cup ricotta cheese. Bake at 400F for 20 minutes in a covered pan.

Chapter 10: The Common Mistakes

A person who is starting a diet for the very first time will find it difficult to stick to the diet. This section covers the common mistakes that are made by people all over the world.

Consuming extra fat

When you start a diet for the very first time, you will see that you will need to cut down on the fat that is harmful to your health. This does not mean that you cut down on the fat that you need to consume. You have to control yourself from starving yourself. You have to ensure that you consume carbohydrates and proteins in the right amounts. When you are on a diet remember that the calories are important and you have to ensure that you consume enough of these calories.

Too much starch

It is true that you need to consume carbohydrates when you are on a diet. This does not mean that you consume every carbohydrate since you will need to cut down on the glycemic content in the carbohydrates. You will need to stop consuming carbohydrates with too much starch in them since they do not help you with losing weight or with staying healthy.

Too many fruits

You may be surprised at this statement since you have been told to consume a lot of fruit. It is true that fruits contain minerals and nutrients and it is important that you consume pieces of fruit. But, too much is always bad for you. Be sure to keep everything in moderation

Gorging on protein bars

Everybody knows that protein is extremely important for the human body since it helps in repairing any tissues and any harm that you may have caused to your body internally. This does not mean that you consume protein bars as your primary source of protein. Real protein obtained through whole foods such as meats and nuts are the sources where you should be getting most of your protein.

Not consuming enough food

This is a mistake that every diet rookie makes. People believe that you have to stop eating if you are looking to weight. You will need to live only on water and on fruit juices in order to lose all the unwanted fat in your body. This is not the right way since you will be starving yourself, which is an extremely bad idea. You have to ensure that you eat the right amount of food at the right time. Make sure that you stick to the schedule. It is one thing to be at a caloric deficit in order to lose weight, but it is a completely different and detrimental thing to be at a daily nutritional deficit.

You have to ensure that you do not make these rookie mistakes since you have to keep yourself healthy. If you find yourself making any of these mistakes, stop and start over again. You have to ensure that you keep motivating yourself in order to succeed at maintaining clean eating habits.

Chapter 11: Detox for a Head Start

A single utterance of the word "Detox" is enough to strike fear and dread into the hearts of even the strong-willed. I am sure you have probably heard of or even tried one of the many Hollywood-endorsed cleanse programs. Some of which, verge on cruel and unusual. Well, it doesn't have to be this way! Whether you want to dive head first into the clean eating lifestyle or you are just feeling it out while making small but meaningful changes in your life, a simple lemon water detox is a great way to start. Each morning when you wake or each night before you go to sleep, have a mug of hot water with the juice of half a lemon squeezed in. I add a drip of honey for a little sweetness and extra antiseptic properties.

The benefits of this miracle elixir are numerous. For example, lemons contain potassium which is helpful in lowering blood pressure, reducing inflammation and strengthening capillaries. The high concentration of vitamin C found in lemons aids in immune support, decreases the appearance of wrinkles, and is useful to manage stress. Sipping hot lemon water has been shown to help prevent and shorten the cold virus and improve digestive health by relieving symptoms of nausea, heartburn, and constipation. Lemon juice encourages the liver to increase production of bile, an acid required for digestion and the effective elimination of waste from the body. Using lemon water as a cleanse for your liver has been proven extremely effective. For weight loss, you can rely on the lemon's content of pectin fiber. Fiber slows the digestive process, thereby reducing food cravings and leaving you feeling fuller for a longer period of time after meals.

Lemons can help regulate the pH of the body, as well. Research has shown that cancer cells thrive in acidic environments. The large majority of processed fast food and junk foods are highly acidic when metabolized in the body causing the pH to shift into acidity and providing cancer cells the perfect setting in which to grow. The whole foods you will consume during your clean eating journey such as fruit, vegetables, tofu, soybeans, nuts, seeds and legumes are all alkaline-promoting. Lemons and other citrus fruits with their alkalinity hold underneath their waxy flesh the ability to prevent cancer cells from flourishing and reduce the symptoms of rheumatoid arthritis.

In tandem with the warm lemon water at bed, you will want to be mindful of your water intake throughout the day. The rule of thumb is to drink – at minimum – half of your body weight in ounces. So, if you weigh 150 lbs., you are going to want to ingest at least 75 ounces per day. This calculation is for routine tasks. The amount of water your body needs to simply function on a normal level. Staying properly hydrated is an essential part of living a healthy lifestyle. An adequate intake of water will result in less fatigue and increased focus.

Are you one of those types who doesn't care too much for the taste of water, or lack thereof? The solution to that little problem is an easy one. Just squeeze a bit of citrus in! Or better yet, make your own flavored water infused with fresh fruit. Personally, I believe that making your water a bit more interesting and desirable will lead to an increased intake. Plus, you will be receiving the benefits of whichever combination of fruits, vegetables and herbs you include as well.

Some of my favorite mash-ups are as follows:

- Lemon, strawberry, and basil

- Blueberry, orange, and ginger

- Citrus, cucumber, and mint

- Strawberry, lime, and cucumber

- Grapefruit with rosemary

- Blueberry and lavender

- Honeydew and raspberry

- Mango, coconut, and lime

Most commonly, mason jars are used to store fruit-infused water but any sealed container would do. Simply stick it in the fridge overnight and enjoy on the go! Feel free to make a few in advance, if you would like.

Chapter 12: Eat the Rainbow

Nature has a pretty creative way of marking by color the benefits of its fruit. I challenge you to spend a week experimenting with different colors. Spend each day contemplating the infinite options and amazing rewards of each color! Try out new foods and different recipes. In the passages that follow, we will take a journey through the colors of the rainbow. Everything your body needs is right at your fingertips and color-coded, at that! Just take a look around. The clean eating movement has us finally realizing that modern conveniences seem to sometimes get in the way of consuming what nature has so simply and generously provided. Whether you are fully committed to a clean lifestyle or you simply want to cure what ails you, look to these colorful fruits and vegetables.

Red fruits and vegetables such as watermelon, cranberries, cherries, tomatoes, radishes, beets, and red peppers contain a significant amount of beta-carotene, or vitamin A. They are also chock full of fiber, antioxidants, lycopene, and vitamin C. Free radicals, heart disease and cancer all shudder in the presence of red foods! A diet rich in these can offer increased gastrointestinal health and joint support.

Foods like carrots, tangerines, apricots, mangos, pumpkin, and sweet potatoes all have something in common and that is beta-cryptoxanthin and beta-carotene. These nutrients support eyesight as well as facilitating a healthy immunity in order to ward off infections and disease. The anti-inflammatory properties of orange foods are also essential for joint and respiratory health.

Aside from the sheer cheeriness and intense flavor of yellow fruits and vegetables like pineapples, lemons, pears, squash, tomatoes, and peppers, you will benefit from their carotenoids and bioflavonoids. Carotenoids are antioxidants that give our immune systems a serious boost and help to protect against heart and retinal disease. A powerful mix of vitamins C and A, potassium, and lycopene are packed into these fantastic yellow packages.

Green foods will be your best friend on this journey, I would say. Your body will love you for going green with these superfoods and will reward you handsomely. Dark leafy greens such as kale, spinach, or beet greens by calorie are probably the most concentrated source of nutrition of any food group delivering to your temple a myriad of minerals, vitamins, and phytonutrients. The list of benefits to consuming at least three servings of leafy greens per day is a mile long. It includes omega-3 fats and minerals such as iron, calcium, magnesium, and potassium. They are crammed with vitamins K, C, E, and B. They also come equipped with phytonutrients like beta-carotene, zeaxanthin, and lutein all protecting your cells and eyes from age-related damage.

Vitamin K is responsible for regulating blood clotting, protects against osteoporosis, and reduces inflammation. A helpful tip when preparing greens high in this vitamin is to remember that it is fat soluble. Be sure to cook or dress your greens with olive oil to get a double punch of vitamins and unsaturated fats. The high level of calcium and fiber found in these type of vegetables is essential for bones and teeth as well as healthy digestion and sustainable energy.

Blue and purple are usually lumped together, as the variations of color are produced by phytochemicals called anthocyanins and resveratrol. Foods rich in these colors have been hailed as antioxidant superfoods for a good reason. They are full of anti-inflammatory and anti-carcinogenic properties, destroying free radicals left and right. They can lower cholesterol and the risk of Alzheimer's disease, diabetes, and obesity. Purple foods also contain quercetin, lutein, and vitamin C for our health and longevity. A few foods that belong to this superhero class are olives, elderberries, purple carrots, plums, and figs.

A common mistake with the rainbow mentality is that we often forget about the importance of consuming food that is white. For example, the nutrients found in foods like cauliflower, jicama, garlic, ginger, parsnips, turnips, and fennel all boast anti-tumor and weight loss properties. They also contain sulfur which is essential for a healthy and detoxified liver.

 Another common mistake would be overlooking foods that are black, for they probably contain more anti-oxidants than anything of lighter color. They contain a higher concentration of pigmentation which is attributed to the anthocyanins found in these types of foods. Anthocyanins are powerful phytonutrients responsible for reducing the risk of heart disease, diabetes, and certain cancers. Try mixing some black chia seeds, black beans, black tea, black lentils, or shiitake mushrooms into your new rainbow diet!

The benefits of brown foods should be addressed, as well. Ancient and whole grains like gluten-free and gut friendly millet, fiber rich freekeh, bulgur that is full of manganese for bone health, kamut which contains the immune boosting mineral selenium, and farro that can stabilize blood sugar and lower cholesterol. Another miracle grain is gluten-free Amaranth which originates from South America and aids in tissue growth and repair. It is helpful to remember that whole grains can go rancid very quickly due to the natural oils. They can be stored in an airtight container for up to six months in a dark, cool place like a pantry or refrigerator.

Chapter 13: Portion Control and Awareness

One last thing to keep in mind on your journey is portion control. Some frightening statistics from the USDA have emerged after researchers evaluated typical serving portions at various takeout restaurants. They found that in the case of pasta, servings exceeded the standard suggestion by 480%. Cookies topped the charts at seven times the recommended serving size.

Your first order of business is to brush up on your food label reading prowess to be able to discern the correct serving size. This is the amount recommended by government agencies such as the USDA, the Department of Health and Human Services, and the Dietary Guidelines for Americans.

Another simple suggestion that could save you from overeating is taking the time to measure accurately. It may seem tedious at first but every little bit adds up. If you are truly putting all of your effort into clean eating, a little oversight or slip-up could really set you back. If you do not have immediate access to a measuring cup or spoon, familiarize yourself with the general serving suggestions of most major food groups and relate that to everyday objects which can be easily remembered and called upon for reference. For example, a 3 oz. portion of cooked meat is roughly the same size as a deck of playing cards. 1 cup would be about the size of a tennis ball and an ounce would be like a domino.

Change the way you serve your food, as well. If you cook for multiple people or a family, portion out servings onto individual plates instead of eating family-style at the table. An additional piece of advice that would help keep control over portions and also make life a little more convenient is to pre-portion meals and snacks. All too often, we sit on the couch with a bag of chips and a bowl full of salsa and just go to town without realizing how much we are actually consuming. Plenty of people just go through the motions and mindlessly snack. When you learn to view food as fuel, you will realize that your body actually only requires a portion of what you had previously been ingesting. Purchase some portion control containers or small zip-lock baggies then go ahead and divide all of your snacks for the week. That way, you can grab and go and really feel good about your decision.

When eating out, remain conscious of portions. It is a little easier to keep an eye on that type of thing at home when you have full control over the ingredients and preparation. When you leave that power in someone else's hands, you have to make some adjustments on your end. The sheer amount of food that restaurants dole out is alarming. The only options are to either leave half of it behind to be thrown away, take it home with you and more than likely forget about it in the refrigerator, or split an entrée with someone.

Conclusion

This book has provided you with great detail about what clean eating is all about. Let us make a checklist of all that we have learnt so far shall we?

1. No Paleo, crash or Juice diets
2. Only consume unrefined food
3. Make sure that you eat healthy!

You have to remember that when you are on a 'diet', you usually have to avoid consuming all the foods you love. You will also need to give up desserts if you need to lose your calories. However, this does not happen when you eat clean. Make sure that you go natural with all your food and also get enough exercise and rest!

You have been given delicious recipes for clean eating and have also been given a sample plan that you can follow for three days. If you ensure that you follow this diet, you will be able to keep yourself healthy and fit. You will also be able to lose weight without any extra effort. Make sure that you stay true to the plan. Clean eating is not really a diet. It is a lifestyle change- a healthy one at that! It is about maintain the appropriate nutritional value that will feed your body what it really needs in order to operate at maximum efficiency!

Let your body work its magic! Thank you!

Ketogenic Diet:

Low-Carb, High Fat Diet Done Properly For Real Weight Loss!

2nd Edition

By reading this document, the reader agrees that under no circumstances are we responsible for any losses, direct or indirect, which are incurred as a result of the use of information contained within this document, including, but not limited to, —errors, omissions, or inaccuracies.

Introduction

Thank you for choosing this book "Ketogenic Diet: Low-Carb, High Fat Diet Done Properly For Real Weight Loss!"

In this book you will learn everything that you need to know about the Ketogenic diet and the lifestyle changes that you can adapt to achieve your weight and fitness goals. This isn't one of those glossy books that promise weight reduction within no time. It will take some serious time and commitment from you to actually make any difference. So, be prepared to make a few changes if you really want this diet to be of any use.

The concept of Ketogenic diet is quite simple. This is a low-carb and a high fat diet. When this diet is followed properly, you will be pleasantly surprised. So, resist your temptations, put in some effort and give this book a thorough reading to lead a happier and a much healthier life. Happy reading!

Chapter 1: All About the Ketogenic Diet

A Ketogenic diet is a low carbohydrate diet where the ketones that are produced by the liver are used as a source of energy. It is also known as the Keto diet or the low-carb and high fat diet. Whenever we consume food that contains carbohydrates, it is immediately converted into glucose and insulin by our body. Glucose is a molecule that is readily converted into energy hence it is chosen over other sources. Meanwhile, insulin is produced by our body to process the glucose present in the blood stream. Since our body is using up all the glucose, it becomes the primary source of energy while fats is just stored up. An average person's diet is high in carbohydrates which implies that the main source of energy is glucose.

When there is a reduction in the intake of carbs, the body is induced into ketosis. Ketosis occurs naturally when the intake of food is low to aid in our survival. In this state, the body produces ketones and are used as a source of energy.

The general idea of the Ketogenic diet is to force the body into a state of ketosis. This is achieved by reducing the intake of carbohydrates and not just by starving the body of calories. Furthermore, when there is an increase in the intake of fats and decrease in the carbs consumed, the body starts burning up the ketones to maintain the required level of energy.

Fast facts about the Ketogenic diet

The following are the facts that you need to know to get a better understanding of this diet:

It is designed to induce a state of ketosis.

Like the name suggests, this diet is designed to induce the body into a state of ketosis by reducing the consumption of carbohydrates. Primarily, the body's source of fuel is carbs and the main source of energy is the easily convertible glucose. When the supply of glucose is restricted, the body moves towards making use of another source of energy which is fat. A normal Ketogenic diet would consist of 70% fats, 20% of proteins and about 5% of carbs.

The primary source of fuel is fat

What we consume, be it fats or carbohydrates, are metabolized and stored by the body. Carbohydrates are broken down into glucose and stored in the muscles and liver, whereas fats are broken down into triglycerides and stored as adipose tissues or body fat. Glucose and triglycerides are both sources of energy. In keto diet, as the body is in ketosis, the fats will be the primary source of fuel and energy. Of course, there is still a need to consume protein.

Low carbs signify low energy

Reducing the intake of carbs will not help you with your exercise regime. When the store of glucose in the body is gradually depleted, it becomes increasingly difficult to exercise. This is why all the endurance sports require the athletes to consume energy drinks and other substitutes. In following the ketogenic diet, the depleted glucose is replaced by ketones and gradually gets the body to get used to burning fat efficiently.

Watch out for high cholesterol

In keto diet, the body starts burning fat to generate energy. Consequently, you might end up with high cholesterol. Cholesterol, a fatty substance, is naturally produced in the body and also found in the food we eat. The increased consumption of foods with LDL cholesterol or bad cholesterol clogs the arteries and causes heart diseases. To counter this, lots of fiber and good fats are highly recommended.

Read food labels and pay attention to the nutrient content

The keto diet requires carb consumption of 50 grams per day or less. In order to achieve this, you will have to start reading the food labels carefully. Most dairy products are high in protein as well as carbohydrates. This also applies to some of the fruits, nuts, legumes and even vegetables. Be wise in your food choices as you commit yourself to this diet.

Carbohydrate cheats

This diet is a real challenge because all the food we eat on a daily basis is mostly made of carbohydrates. Spaghetti Bolognese will not be the same without the spaghetti, right? This is where carbohydrate cheats come in. You need to find low-carb alternatives like replacing rice with cauliflower rice or zucchini ribbons instead of pasta. Almond flour and peanut flour are healthy as well. Consider this, a portion of $1/4^{th}$ cup of cooked brown rice or even one boiled sweet potato consists of almost as much as 12.5 grams of carbs. Research each food's carbohydrate content and compare them as you go along this diet.

Side effects to look out for

Aside from the desired effect of losing weight, there are also some side effects to be aware of in the keto diet. These are nausea, headache, lethargy and sleepiness. This diet can be tough on both the body and the mind. Some people have had cognitive reduction (fogginess, increased confusion etc.) and mood swings. A combination of these symptoms is referred to as the Keto flu. These side effects are on a case to case basis and not the same for everyone. However, it is best to seek professional advice or consult your dietician before and during the diet for some healthy guidelines.

Nutritional deficits must be addressed effectively

The diet would make your body get rid of sodium, potassium and water content drastically resulting to the Keto flu. While the body is capable of adjusting to any minor changes in the level of electrolytes, an increase in the water intake will cause an imbalance in the electrolytes. Water is good but we do not want to spoil the harmony of electrolytes in the body. Also, steer clear of sweetened drinks.

Bad breath

This diet will definitely give you a bad breath. Ketones are produced when fat is burned for energy instead of carbohydrates. The ketones provide energy to the brain. With all that burning of excessive fat, the amount of ketones produced is also high. One way the body gets rid of excess ketones is through breath, hence the bad breath. Since the root cause of this problem isn't deficiency in oral health, you can't get rid of this problem by brushing or flossing. The only practical way to get rid of it is by consuming more carbs which will be in contradictory with what the keto diet promotes. A temporary solution would be breath mints.

Chapter 2: Myths About Fat Consumption

Fats aren't that bad. In fact, consumption of fats is good for your body. It is the mindset towards fat that has given it a bad reputation. In this chapter we will take a look at some myths about consumption of fats that have caused unnecessary fear.

Myth#1 - Consumption of fat will make you fat.

This isn't true. The fat in our ordinary diet is different from the one that is stored in our body. The body takes a lot more time to digest fat than any other nutrient source and the feeling of fullness comes from the nutrients. Technically, the consumption of fat would help cut down on calorie intake which is actually good. Fat is a nutrient just like proteins and carbohydrates. It helps in the absorption of vitamins and when broken down into fatty acids it also sustains the brain. So consumption of fats is quintessential for your good health.

Still, eating fatty foods must be in moderation. Eating too much of it together with refined carbohydrates can lead to unnecessary weight gain.

Myth#2 - There are healthy and unhealthy fats.

It is a general misconception that fats are only of two kinds: the good ones and the bad ones where trans fat and saturated fats are the bad fats while unsaturated ones are good. Well, the distinction between these fats is more complicated. Fats are of seven kinds. The type of fats ranging from the most to the least healthy are: Omega 3 fats, monounsaturated fats, polyunsaturated fats, saturated fats, medium chain triglycerides, Omega 6 fatty acids and then Trans fat. What you should focus on is eating fats that fall in the top of the above mentioned list.

Myth#3 - Trans fat isn't all that bad.

Even small amounts of trans fat will shorten our life span because they get accumulated in the body. Bacteria are incapable of digesting trans fats thus it is added to some processed foods to increase its shelf life. Whenever you consume trans fat, the body does not digest it so it ends up lining and clogging the body's arteries and liver. As a result, there is an increased risk of developing various coronary diseases, cardio vascular diseases as well as damage to arteries.

Myth#4- Foods labeled with 0 grams trans fat are perfectly safe.

Avoiding trans fat at any cost is a must in this diet. While buying food products, do pay some heed to their labels. If per serving a product contains less than 0.4 grams of trans fat, then it legally can be listed as 0 grams trans fat. Let's say you bought it and end up consuming four servings of such food products. Computing that, your consumption of trans fat is 2 grams. This might not seem much, but it can definitely make you sick. A really effective way to detect foods that contain trans fat is by reading their labels carefully. *Partially hydrogenated oil* in the ingredients used also contains trans fat, avoid it as well.

Myth#5- For better health, consume less saturated fats.

For years, we have been blaming saturated fats for all the cardiovascular diseases. In truth, saturated fats are cardiovascular neutral meaning they neither cause nor help these diseases. People who consume a lot meats and food rich in saturated fats are at a higher risk when compared to those who don't or eat less of such foods. Still, the same can be said if the saturated fats are replaced with processed and refined carbs with added sugars in a person's diet. Even if you avoid greasy bacon for breakfast and eat sugary cereal, the risk of heart diseases is the same. A diet that is full of refined carbs is as bad as a diet full of saturated fats from meats and various other sources. It's still a matter of making healthy food choices.

Myth#6- Full fat dairy products are bad for the health.

The fat in dairy products is absorbed differently from the fats in other foods. People who consume full fat dairy products in fact are less likely to be overweight than others who do not consume the same. Their risk to high blood pressure and type-2 diabetes is significantly lower and more likely to live longer compared to those who consume the low fat dairy varieties.

Myth#7 - The healthiest of oils is olive oil.

Olive oil indeed is very healthy. Unfortunately, when heated up, its healthy monounsaturated fats are converted into saturated fats and even to trans fat. Going back to myth #2, these fats are at the bottom of the healthy list. Healthier alternatives are peanut oil, avocado and sesame oils.

Myth#8- Salad dressings are unhealthy

Dietary fiber is very important to the body. It is required in absorbing the nutrients in the food. Completely avoiding fat in salad dressings is no good. In forgoing the dressings or making use of fat free dressing like vinegar, you might be cutting on the calories but it really won't do your body any good.

Myth#9- Cardio can burn fat.

There's a grain of truth in this statement but this does not happen immediately. There's around 1000 calories stored in the liver that are easy to burn. This reserve needs to be burned out before the body can start breaking down fat for fuel. Even an hour of cardio does not burn 1000 calories. Don't worry about how to burn through the calorie store in your body, every little amount of exercise you do will bring you a step closer to achieving your goal.

Chapter 3: Benefits of Ketogenic Diet

Health professionals demonize diets that are low in carb and high in fat content across the world. It was a popular belief that such diets would exponentially increase the chances of individuals of beings susceptible to heart diseases, all due to the high content of fat. Well, this isn't the case these days. Since the beginning of this century a lot of research has been conducted and most of the results point out that keto diets are much better when compared to the others. A low-carb diet not only helps in shedding weight but it also helps in improving the overall health and correcting major health risks like cholesterol.

Let us take a look at ten benefits of the Ketogenic diet:

Reduction in appetite (not in a bad way)

The most difficult side effect to cope with while dieting is hunger. This is the most leading reason why a lot of people give up on their diets. An advantage of a low-carb diet is it aids in the reduction of your appetite. Once you start cutting down on carbohydrate intake and replacing it with protein and fat, the amount of calories you consume will also be reduced. The decrease in carbs intake in turn decreases a person's appetite.

Facilitates in more weight loss

One of the simplest and the most effective way to shed the extra kilos is by cutting down on carbs. Studies show that a person who is on a low-carb diet when compared to a low fat diet is bound to reduce weight more rapidly. One reason is that the excess water present in the body is removed. Once the insulin level in the body is reduced and the kidneys start getting rid of the sodium, there is a noticeable weight loss in the first week.

The keto diet is observed to be very effective for the first six months or so. It would remain effective if maintained as a lifestyle. Eating low-carb is a diet and a way of life at the same time. In accepting and believing this, the process would be much easier to adjust to. Always find ways to accommodate healthier options for carbohydrates into your diet once you have achieved your ideal weight. It wouldn't be an exaggeration to say that a low-carb diet will definitely help in rapid weight loss, provided you follow it regularly and consistently.

Abdominal fat will be shed.

All the fat present in the body is not the same. Health risks vary depending upon the location and concentration of fats in the body. They are mostly stored either under our skin as a layer of fat or in the abdominal cavity. Visceral fat tends to accumulate around the organs that may result in inflammation and obstruction of insulin making it one of the prominent causes of metabolism dysfunction.

A low-carb diet is very effective in getting rid of this harmful fat in the viscera and abdominal cavity. Adapting to the Ketogenic lifestyle reduces the risk of heart diseases and even type-2 diabetes over a period of time.

Reduction of triglycerides

Triglycerides are molecules of fat present in the body from the breaking down of fats. An increase in the amount of triglycerides in the blood likewise increases the risk of heart diseases. This increase of triglycerides is attributed to the consumption of carbohydrates specifically simple sugar fructose. The obvious effect of following a low-carb diet is the reduction in triglycerides levels in the blood. Oppositely, a low-fat diet increases triglycerides levels in the blood.

The amount of triglycerides is directly proportional to the amount of carbs that you consume. Furthermore, the higher the triglyceride, the higher is the risk of heart diseases.

Improvement in the level of good cholesterol

High-density lipoprotein (HDL) is often referred to as the good cholesterol. Technically, it is incorrect to refer to it as cholesterol since all the cholesterol molecules have the same composition. HDL and LDL are the lipoproteins that help in the transportation of cholesterol in the blood stream.

Low-density lipoprotein (LDL) is responsible for carrying the cholesterol molecules to the liver and the rest of the body whereas the high-density lipoprotein (HDL) is responsible for carrying the cholesterol molecules away from the body, either for reuse or excretion.

A higher level of HDL means that the risk of heart diseases is lower. One of the most efficient ways of increasing HDL is by the consumption of healthy fats. Low-carb diets recommend this as well. It comes as no surprise that the HDL levels of individuals who follow the Ketogenic diet are high when compared to those who follow a low-fat diet. The ratio of triglycerides and LDL is also another indicator of risk for heart diseases. The higher this ratio is the greater is the risk of heart diseases. Reduction in the level of triglycerides and the simultaneous increase in the levels of HDL can be achieved by following a low-carb diet.

Reduction in the level of both insulin and blood sugar

The carbs that we consume are broken down into simple sugars in the digestive system. Simple sugars enter our blood stream and increase the level of blood sugar. High levels of blood sugars is extremely toxic to the body thus the body produces a hormone called insulin. Insulin helps the cells to bring glucose to the cells either to burn it as energy or store it. Normally, this insulin response is the body's way of reducing a spike in the blood sugar to prevent any further damage to the body.

One of the most common problems plaguing mankind is diabetes. This is a metabolic disease where the pancreas is not producing enough insulin or the body cells are not reacting properly to the insulin present in the blood. One type of this is the type-2 diabetes where the body fails to generate sufficient insulin to help in the breakdown of blood sugars in the blood. A simple solution is to cut down on carbs consumption. There will be no more need to generate more insulin thus, both the blood sugar levels and insulin levels decrease. If you are on medication to reduce your blood sugar and want to follow the Ketogenic diet, consult your doctor first because the dosage of your medication might need to be adjusted for the prevention of hypoglycemia.

To sum it up, reduce the amount of carbs you consume to reduce the blood sugar and insulin levels.

Lowered blood pressure

Hypertension or having an abnormally high levels of blood pressure is a leading factor in causing heart diseases and other diseases like kidney failure and damage to eye sight. The Ketogenic diet will help in controlling the levels of blood pressure and reducing the risk of the above-mentioned diseases.

Promotes treatment of metabolic syndrome

Metabolic syndrome is a medical condition associated with a high risk of diabetes and heart diseases. Its symptoms are elevated blood pressure and sugar levels, abdominal obesity, high levels of triglycerides and low levels of HDL. These symptoms when not kept in check, will eventually lead to various heart diseases and even type-2 diabetes as well. Successfully fight and reverse all these symptoms by following the Ketogenic diet. Disappointingly, the government as well as key health organizations still recommend a low fat diet when these symptoms can be effectively reversed by following a low-carb diet.

An improved LDL levels

Low Density Lipoprotein (LDL) carries the cholesterol molecules to the liver and the rest of the body. Research shows that people with high levels of LDL are often more prone to heart diseases. Recent studies show that it is important to identify the type of LDL present in the body because not all of them are equal. To determine the type of LDL, the criteria is based on its size. Individuals who have small particles of LDL are more prone to heart diseases than the ones who have large particles of it. Following a low-carb diet increases the size of the LDL particles while its number floating in the blood stream are reduced.

Keto diet have two positive results on LDL particles: 1. its size increases making them benign and 2. its concentration in the blood stream decreases.

Helps in treating several disorders of the brain

FACT: The brain needs a constant supply of glucose. A part of the brain is equipped for burning glucose only. This is why our liver produces glucose even out of protein when we don't consume any carbs. Fortunately, a major portion of our brain can burn ketones as well and these are produced either when our body is being starved or when the carb intake has been reduced. This is the mechanism that has been made use of during the Ketogenic diet. It has proven to be effective in treating epilepsy, especially in children who do not respond to any other form of treatment. A study shows that when children suffering from epilepsy were made to follow the Ketogenic diet, there was about 50% decrease in seizures.

Of late, studies on diets based on low or no carbohydrates consumption in correlation to brain disorders like Alzheimer's and Parkinson's are being conducted.

Chapter 4: Side Effects of Over-consumption of Carbs

A healthy and balanced diet is the key to good health. Overeating creates an imbalance leading to a number of nasty after effects. The calories stored in the body increase exponentially leading to obesity and other problems related to it. Stress eating is a common scenario. We tend to crave carbohydrates in times of stress that later on becomes a bad eating habit. The following are the side effects of consuming too much refined and processed carbohydrates:

Blood sugar levels imbalance

Like mentioned earlier, too much of anything is not beneficial for the body. Too much refined carbohydrates in particular messes with the blood sugar levels. When you eat a slice of cake with frosting on it, it increases the levels of insulin in the body and results in the storage of glucose. Insulin balances out blood sugar levels and keeps them in a normal range. As blood sugar levels rise, the pancreas secretes more insulin. If the body does not produce enough insulin or the cells are resistant to the effects of insulin, hyperglycemia develops and causes long-term complications when not addressed. These imbalances in the blood stream tend to disrupt the functioning of the human body as a whole.

Weight gain

Consumption of foods high in saturated fats or even carbs will result in unnecessary weight gain. Foods that are rich in refined carbs lead to weight gain because they are mostly empty calories that lead to more carb craving. There are a couple of healthy sources to get your carbohydrates requirement like fruits and vegetables. So instead of picking a bowl of pasta, opt for your favorite protein. Find alternatives for carbs and stick to those for a healthier life.

Functioning of the brain

Brain fatigue or brain fog is an episode of mental confusion brought about by many factors, one of which is diabetes. It is characterized by confusion, a lack of focus, poor memory recall, and reduced mental acuity. Fluctuating glucose levels in the blood can cause short term brain fatigue symptoms.

Chapter 5: Things to Consider

Ketogenic diet is not just a diet but a lifestyle choice. It is not a fad. This diet is backed by research that shows the manner in which the metabolism of our body changes when we cut back on the consumption of carbohydrates and increase the fats consumed. There are certain things that you will have to consider before you get started with this diet and this chapter talks about these in detail.

Seek professional help

It will be helpful if you can consult a professional or a health care practitioner who can help you chalk out a proper meal plan. It will also help you avoid mistakes along the way and ensure that your body is not deprived of any important macro-nutrients. Getting started on a diet is not really difficult when you know what you are supposed to do and what you can and cannot eat. Figuring out all this on your own might prove to be a challenge. The very idea of going through this tedious process might be a turn off for a lot of people. Individuals who are suffering epilepsy should consider the diet with their nutritionist before they get started with it. Even if you are on any medication, do consult your doctor before giving this diet a go, especially when it comes to children.

Blood tests are important

Get a complete blood work done before starting on this diet to ensure that you aren't suffering from any condition that you might not be aware of. Consult your physician once you get your results and seek approval to get on with this diet. Some suggested tests to get done are lipid profile, thyroid panel, inflammatory markers, full blood count and tests for liver/kidney functioning. If you suffer from fatigue then you can add a little of B12 supplements to your meal to get rid of anemia.

There's no rush

Take it easy, especially during the initial stages of this diet. There's no need to cut down your carbohydrate intake straight away. Gradually decrease carbohydrate intake over a period of few weeks. Some doctors even recommend a fast to ensure that your body goes into ketosis easily, but do not do this if you haven't done it before. Consult a doctor first.

Select the timing

It might not be the most ideal time for the implementation of this diet if you are busy (physically, emotionally or even psychologically) for two reasons. The first one is that you will be stressed about cooking with certain restrictions. Meals and the method of preparation employed will take a little getting used. It will be like setting yourself up for failure when you are off to a shaky start. Second, it will be challenging, not impossible but it will take a toll on you adding more to the stress you are already in.

Let us take the instance of a cancer patient. If the patient has started with chemotherapy, it is not advisable to follow this diet immediately. It will be extremely difficult because most of the drugs used in chemotherapy have a glucose base. This means that the level of glucose in the body will be high and ketosis will be non-existent. It would be helpful instead to finishing chemotherapy, maintaining a good metabolic balance by exercising and eating balanced food rich in nutrients. Take sufficient time to let the body cope with all the medication. For an athlete, select an appropriate time to put this diet into action. It does not make sense to go on a keto diet on competition season as it will mean giving up on carbs and a reduction in the energy produced by the body. The body's adaptation to this lifestyle can range from a week to a month. This is a risk you shouldn't take when the conditions are not favorable.

Plan ahead

This diet can't be done randomly. Research and read on Ketogenic diets to be equipped on meals and all the necessary requirements. Plan ahead, make a list, and get some grocery shopping done. Depending upon your body type, there will also be some foods that might not provide you sufficient nourishment. You will also need to make a list of things you might be allergic to. Take into consideration some food sensitivity symptoms connected to consumption of some food products like an increased heart rate after a meal, constipation, mood swings and other digestive problems. One good thing about following the Ketogenic diet is that most of the products that are likely to cause allergic reactions like wheat or even peanuts are mostly eliminated. Only when you have a better idea of what all you can consume without having to face any unpleasantness will you be able to achieve the optimal results from this diet.

Social life

Once you start this diet, commit to follow it to see some substantial improvement. This means that you will have to stick to your diet even while eating out, socializing and travelling as well. This might be a little difficult in the beginning. You don't want your diet to clash with any major events that are coming up in your life like a birthday party or even a vacation. A little bit of planning and mental toughening is required. A lot of people might comment about the foods that you consume. Be ready for a verbal onslaught of gasps and sighs. It is normal that people would comment when they see you gorging on fat and protein while ignoring the carbs. Ignore all the advice you get from others apart from the one given to you by your doctor.

Essentials

Ketone or glucose meters and even weighing scales are essentials aside from the food. Weigh out your foods before you consume them. This extra effort will go a long way for the diet to work properly. Some kitchen equipment like a good blender, steamer, non-toxic fry pans, and proper storage containers when you want to freeze any of the food cooked are also recommended to be on hand.

Keep going, don't give up

You will need to keep going even after achieving the optimal state of ketosis. One way in which you can do this is by finding a constant stream of recipes and ideas that can be incorporated into your diet to avoid the boredom of repetition. Ensure that your source of information is Ketogenic friendly. Educate yourself and beware of all the self styled experts on the web doling out advice.

Chapter 6: What to Eat

It is good that you are interested in trying out the Ketogenic diet. But when you have got no idea about the food products that you should and shouldn't consume, following a diet would be an absolute nightmare. In this chapter, provided is a comprehensive list of the things that you can and cannot eat. Being conscious of what you eat is the first step of ensuring that the diet is going to be effective. If you are suffering from any condition that causes imbalances in the levels of blood sugar in your body, consult your doctor before starting the diet.

Read through this chapter carefully.

Fats and oils

The major portion of your calorie intake will come from this category on a daily basis. Fats are essential for the functioning of your body but these can prove to be incredibly dangerous when the wrong types of fat are consumed. Balance out Omega 3 and Omega 6 fatty foods. Trout, salmon, tuna and even shellfish can help maintain the required balance of Omega 3 in your daily diet. Supplements are recommended to people with allergic reactions to seafood or have a dislike to seafood. Fish oil supplements maintain the required amount of Omega 3 in the body.

For saturated and monounsaturated fats, consume butter, macadamia nuts, egg yolks and avocado as well. These products have chemical stability and don't cause any inflammation. Combine fats and oils together and add this to your meals in different ways. You can make sauces or even dressings for your salads or just add a dollop of butter to your meats. Avoid hydrogenated fats as well as trans fats. Steer clear of products like margarine. Studies show that the consumption of such undesirable fats is directly proportional to the risk of heart diseases. Cold pressed oils are the best choice if you are using vegetable oils such as olive oil, soya bean or even sunflower oil. In frying, make use of non hydrogenated oils like beef tallow, ghee or even coconut oil because the smoke point of these oils is usually high allowing for lesser oxidization. This ensures that your body will receive more of the necessary fatty acids. Also, watch the amount of nuts or any seed based food that you eat. These contain Omega 6 and is inflammatory in nature. Eat almonds, walnuts, pine nuts and even some seed-based oils in moderation.

The following are a great source of both oils and fats that you can include in the diet: avocado, beef tallow, chicken fat, macadamia nuts, butter, ghee, mayonnaise and any other non-hydrogenated lard, coconut oil, olive oil, sunflower oil or even peanut oil. If any of the above mentioned products are available in the organic or the grass fed range, choose those instead of the regular ones.

Protein

The variety of produce for you to choose from for meeting the daily requirement of protein is quite varied. Whenever possible opt for the organic or grass fed meats as they are healthier. The list of proteins that you can choose from are:

Fish: Tuna, flounder, mahi mahi, catfish, cod, salmon, snapper, mackerel, trout, halibut, and anything caught in the wild is a safe bet.

Shellfish: Squid, lobster, crabs, scallops, oyster, mussels and clams.

Eggs: Get the free range eggs whenever possible. Consume a whole egg and don't discard the yolk. You can scramble, poach, fry, devil or just boil them.

Meat: Grass fed meets are a better option compared to the steroid injected meats available these days. Beef, veal, goat, lamb and any other game meat are good choices.

Pork: Pork loin, chops and ham are good though watch out for any added sugars when consuming pork.

Poultry: Opt for free-range produce whenever you can. Chicken, duck, quail, and pheasant are the recommended.

Bacon: Whenever you want to consume bacon and sausages, check the labels thoroughly to see that it does not contain any extra filler and is not cured in sugar.

Peanut butter: This can contain Omega 6 and even carbs, so be careful while consuming peanut butter. Other choice is macadamia nut butter.

Vegetables

Vegetables are essential. While following the Ketogenic diet, choose vegetables that are grown above ground like leafy green vegetables. Organic vegetables have additional nutrients when compared to non-organic produce. Some vegetables just don't meet the nutritional cut for this diet. The best type of vegetables need to keep in tune with the basic principle of the Keto diet: they should be low carb. Yes, you guessed it right, dark and leafy vegetables are the best options. Spinach or even kale can be consumed without any second thoughts. The vegetables that you can eat while in keto diet include: avocado, asparagus, broccoli, cauliflower, carrots, celery, green beans, cucumber, garlic, mushrooms, green onions, bell peppers, pickles, dill, romaine lettuce, shallots, snow peas, squash, spinach, kale and tomatoes. Avoid potatoes, sweet potatoes among others.

Dairy Products

Dairy products are an essential part of your diet. Choose the full fat produce. If you can get your hands on raw and organic milk products, you can consume heavy whipping cream, hard and soft cheeses, sour cream and milk. Cheese lovers needn't give up on their love for cheese but don't overeat. Dairy products address your fat and calcium requirements.

Nuts and seeds

Nuts are probably the best way to get rid of all the anti-nutrients present. Do avoid peanuts, since they fall under the category of legumes and legumes are not a part of the Ketogenic diet. Nuts are really good for the health but this does not give you the reason to overeat. You can have almonds, walnuts and macadamia nuts in small quantities. Cashews and pistachios contain more carbs than previously mentioned nuts. Nuts have a high content of Omega 6, so eat in moderate quantities. Instead of regular flour, choose flour made out of nuts and seeds like almond flour and flax seed flour. This gives you the freedom to indulge yourself in guilty pleasures every once in a while while steering clear of the regular flour.

Beverages

Ensure that you are fully hydrated while following the Ketogenic diet because it is diuretic in nature. Be more cautious if you are susceptible to urinary tract infection or bladder pain as well. Keep your body hydrated throughout the day. Drink at least 8 glasses of water and a little more if you can manage to. Keep drinking liquids but avoid anything that has artificial sweeteners, fruit juices or any packaged drinks. Coffee and tea can also be consumed in moderation with very little sugar as much as possible. Stay away from soda and other aerated drinks.

Chapter 7: Five Common Low-carb Mistakes

In this chapter, we will take a look at five rookie mistakes that are committed while dieting and the ways you can avoid them. If you really want your body to enter ketosis in its true sense, then just cutting back on carbs won't do the trick. If you haven't gotten the optimal results after following the Ketogenic diet, then it is more than likely that you have been committing the following mistakes.

Consumption of carbs

There is no proper definition of the term "low-carb." This changes from person to person and even the region they live in. For instance, anything below 100 and 150 grams per day will be considered low in carbs according to the Western standards. A lot of people might even be able to achieve the optimal results even after consuming the above mentioned amount of carbs provided they stayed away from processed foods. Generally, if you keep the consumption of carbs below 50 grams per day, it will help your body to enter ketosis. If you really want your body to enter the full ketosis mode, then even this amount of carbs is undesirable. Experimentation with your diet is the best way to figure out the amount of carbs that you can consume. This means that the sources of carbs become limited and you will have to choose from vegetables and small quantities of fruits.

To make the most of this diet then it is recommended that you limit your carb consumption to less than 50 grams per day.

Consumption of protein

Protein is the main source of energy in this diet. It makes you feel full, reduces your appetite in a good way and it also increases the ability of your body to burn out fat when compared to other micronutrients. To put it simply, the consumption of more protein will help in rapid weight loss. In a low-carb diet, you will still need to mind the amount of protein you are consuming. Eating more protein than what is required by the body will convert amino acids to glucose. Once this happens, your body cannot go into full ketosis. A proper Ketogenic diet should be low in the content of carbohydrates, high in fat and should include moderate amount of proteins. The suitable range for consumption of protein would be anywhere between 1.5 and 2 grams per kilo. Avoid gluconeogenesis, the process of conversion of protein into glucose, and try to keep your consumption of protein within the desired ranges.

Shying away from fat

Most of the calories we consume come from carbs specifically from sugars and various grains. When you stop consuming carbohydrates, a substitute source of energy is necessary. Assuming that low-carb diet goes in hand with low fat diet is a bad idea. The Ketogenic diet restricts the carbs to be replaced with healthy fats. There is no reason to be scared of consuming fats as long as you opt for good fats like Omega 3's and saturated fats.

Replacement of sodium

The mechanism at work that makes the Ketogenic diet a success is the reduction in the level of insulin that is produced in the body.

Insulin is essential for your body because it helps the cells balance glucose, to store fat and signals the kidneys to keep some sodium in the body. In Ketogenic diet, the amount of insulin generated in the body gets reduced wherein the body starts getting rid of sodium along with water. This is why people tend to shed a few kilos within days of following the Keto diet. It is really important that your body has sufficient sodium because it is an electrolyte. One of the main reasons for the failure of this diet would be the reduction in the sodium content present in the body. Its side effects are fatigue, frequent headaches, constipation and even lightheadedness. The best way to avoid this is to add sodium to your diet. Add a little bit of salt to your food. Another way to address this is to consume a cup of broth. You can make a meal out of it as well. Make some light broth, add some lean protein or vegetables and there you have it, a healthy soup.

When you reduce the consumption of carbs, insulin produced is reduced as well. This means the body starts getting rid of sodium as well and might cause a mild deficiency of sodium.

Show some patience

The body is naturally gives preference to burn carbs provided they are available. When you get rid of carbs in your diet, the body will move towards burning fat to generate energy. This adaptation is going to take a few days and during this stage of initiation you might feel a little out of sorts. This is natural and referred to as the low-carb flu. The time taken by your body to fully adapt itself to the burning of fat molecules for the production of energy can take a few weeks. So, be patient and stick to your diet. Let the metabolism of your body get used to this diet. The results generated will be nothing short of miraculous.

Chapter 8: Science Behind the Ketogenic Diet

When it comes to the ketogenic diet, there are some things that work in its favor. This means that the diet will have a positive bearing on your body, which will aid in you losing your excess weight.

Protein intake

The body needs proteins for many purposes. When you consume excess proteins, you end up increasing the metabolic activity in your body. This in turn causes your body to remain slim for long. Proteins are very filling. They will help you feel full without having to eat too much. You will also feel energetic and not feel the need to consume any sugar.

Water break down

Have you heard of water weight? It refers to the weight of the water inside the body. Fat in the body generally stores some water. Once that is freed, the body weight will automatically come down. In the ketogenic diet, your body will start shedding the excess water from the body. The water will also take away with it toxins which will further add to your body's health.

General metabolism

The ketogenic diet helps in setting the body's metabolism in motion. It aids in accelerating the body metabolism and you will feel stronger and fitter within a few days of being on the diet. You might feel lighter as well because the food will not stay in your body for too long. Hence, the ketogenic diet will help you remain stronger and fitter for a long time.

Chapter 9: Mistakes to Avoid with the Diet

Not planning ahead

Without a concrete plan in place will cause you to not take the diet seriously. Create a plan of action and follow through in order to make the diet a lifetime choice. Imagine what would happen if you went to a foreign country without a map. You would get lost and would not enjoy the journey. Similarly, you should plan out your diet and follow through with it. It does not have to be a military level plan; it can be simple yet effective.

Calorie intake

Many people make the mistake of not checking whether they are consuming too many calories in a bid to cut down on the carbs. This end up causing them to go back on their diet's effects on the body. For this, you have to identify the different foods that are full of calories and cut down on them. If you don't know what they are, consider making a list of all the foods that you consume now and then go through each one's calorie content. Surely you will find a few that are highly calorific. Avoid consuming those as much as possible.

Zero nutrition

Another mistake is eating low carb foods and ending up cutting out all the nutrition as well. This is not the right way to go about in any diet. The nutritional content in the food must be quite high with vitamins, minerals and other nutrients to help the body remain strong. This is possible through a list of all the healthy foods to consume and then try to incorporate them as much as possible in your diet. Once you come up with a meal plan, you will find it easy to see what you are consuming and what extra needs to be added in.

Fibrous meals

Fiber is an important part of the diet. Consume as much of it as possible in order to aid in digestion. It is ideal for you to increase its intake if you think you're not consuming enough fiber. Some sources of fiber include vegetables, fruits, nuts and seeds. You can munch on these after a meal and help your body digest food better. You will also feel quite energetic and not have to deal with mood swings.

Munching nuts

It is a great idea for people to munch on nuts, as they are full of essential oils that are great for the body and will keep the joints lubricated. But, it is completely wrong for a person on a low carb diet to consume it as these nuts might cause unnecessary weight gain. It is best for you to avoid consuming them and look at other things as snacking choices. You can, for example, consume cut vegetables such as carrots or beets as they will be sweet and tasty and yet great for your diet.

Not timing it

It is important to time the consumption of carbohydrates. Although you cannot completely eliminate them from your diet, you can time it right to help digest and get it eliminated better. It is best to consume the carbs just before exercising. The body will get a jump-start and will be able to digest the carbs much easily.

No supplements

Many people don't realize that it is important to consume supplements in order to maintain a healthy body. These supplements are full of nutrients that will make the body strong and are also going to help you with your diet. You can take some general supplements such as calcium and vitamin tablets to supplement your diet but you might need more. To know what supplements to consume, visit your doctor and seek advice on what supplements you need. Based on your food habits, he or she will suggest the supplements that you should be consuming.

Being stressed

A lot of unnecessary stress and tension will impact your body negatively. Your mind will make it difficult for you to concentrate on anything, let alone your diet. So it will be quite necessary for you to stop stressing out and relax your mind. Find activities that you can do on a regular basis and reduce your stress levels. You might also have to find out what is causing the stress in the first place and reduce it as much as possible.

Sleeping less

Sleeping less than your normal sleeping hours can also impact your body negatively. It is impossible to be healthy if you stay up late and not get enough sleep. It is best to get at least 8 hours of sleep and without too many disturbances. Make use of some light music to fall asleep or burn a few aroma candles to help you sleep better. You might also have to drain away as much stress and tension before sleeping in order to avail peaceful sleep.

Expecting too much

Expecting too much from your diet is never going to help you. Set reasonable expectations and do not go overboard with what you wish to attain from it. Try to go about it one step at a time. Don't start with the diet the previous day and expect to see positive results the next day. It will take a little time but you will see results for sure. Don't worry if you have gone back a little on the diet. You can always catch up and make the most of it once you take it up seriously.

Too many cheat meals

It is known that the low carb diet allows one cheat meal. These cheat meals are meant to help you stick with the diet. You can have one, once in a while. But, it is important to not get carried away and have too many cheat meals. Some people end up having more than 1 cheat meal a week and simply increase their calorie intake. This might cause you to fall back to your old eating habits. Control yourself as much as possible and set a limit to your cheat meals.

Not exercising

Exercise is a part of any healthy diet. It helps the body lose some of the excess weight and also cut down on the fat cells. If you don't exercise, then you might not be able to lose weight as fast as you can. Sketch out a weight loss plan and follow through it. The exercises don't have to be too rigorous. We will look at a simple exercise plan at the end of this book that will help you come up with your own exercise and weight loss plan.

These are the mistakes to avoid with the low carb diet.

Chapter 10: Some drawbacks and their remedies

There are some drawbacks of the ketogenic diet that you should be aware of before taking it up. These drawbacks are quite normal and will not stay too long.

Frequent urination

When on the low carb or the ketogenic diet, you will feel like urinating too often. This is very common and nothing that you should worry too much about. The diet causes your body to break down the glucose present in your kidney and liver, which might cause a lot of water to release in the body. You have to be prepared to run to the bathroom more often as a result. However, don't assume that drinking less water will help you resolve the issue. There is no correlation between the two and you might not be able to solve the problem. So, don't cut down on the number of glasses of water you gulp down in a day. You should maintain the same, especially if you want the water to further help with your diet.

Bad breath

Bad breath is another major side effect of the ketogenic diet. Many people complain that their breath has worsened and despite brushing their teeth regularly it still smells quite bad. This is mainly because of ketosis. Although this should not be too much of a problem if you brush your teeth thrice and also clean your tongue, you will be able to stave off the bad breath for a long time. You can also consider rinsing your mouth with mouthwash thrice a day. Munching on a few mint or basil leaves will help you maintain fresh breath.

Mood swings

Mood swings are a common side effect of the ketogenic diet. Many people complain about being too grumpy one minute and then normal the next. All of this will cause you to feel uneasy. Try to control your mood by consuming the right foods. Increasing your water intake and also the fiber content in your food will go a long way in helping you stave off the mood swings. You will also feel happy if you sip on some fruit infused water.

Tiredness

Tiredness or fatigue is another complaint that many people have when on the ketogenic diet. Although it is quite common for people on the ketogenic diet to feel tired and out of breath, it is not easy to handle. The excess water that is eliminated from the body will carry with it minerals and salts that are essential for the body. This will cause you to weaken. Therefore, it is important to consume supplements that will help in restoring some of these back into your body. You will feel much more energetic and not feel as dizzy. You can also consume a glass of water to which some salt has been added in. This will help in restoring the salt content in your body and reducing the dizziness.

Headaches

Headaches are a common aspect of the ketogenic diet. This is also mainly caused by the loss of minerals and salts in the body. Some people also complain of having very little energy and possibly flu like symptoms. If you are feeling any of this, then it is obvious that they are caused by the diet. Taking supplements is the best option and also consuming a little extra salt with your diet. In fact, just increasing the water intake will go a long way in helping you restore your energy and reduce the headaches by some margin.

Low sugar

Low sugar levels are common amongst keto dieters. The body will be going through the process of cutting down on the fat in the body and that will cause the sugar levels to reduce as well. It is important for your body to maintain a steady sugar level, especially if you wish to remain energetic. You might crave sweets and chocolates, which can be quite bad for the diet. Do not give into your cravings. As for the weakness, munch on vegetables. It will add in some mild glucose which will not interfere with your diet. The sugar craving will disappear after a while and it is best that you ignore it until your body settles in with the diet.

Constipation

Constipation is another major bodily complaint that most people have when they take up the ketogenic diet. The loss of magnesium and also calcium to some extent will cause you to feel constipated. It will feel like the food is not getting digested so you might experience bloating and uneasiness especially during the initial days of the diet when the body is yet to adjust to it. Constipation can also cause stomachache, which will feel quite uneasy. The best solution is to consume lots of fibrous foods. These foods will help in the bowel movement. You can also consume other foods and supplements that act as mild laxatives and ease bowel movement.

Diarrhea

It is quite interesting to know that some people feel constipated thanks to the ketogenic diet while some others suffer from diarrhea. The intake of too much protein can cause the digestive system to go for a toss. To remedy this issue, you may take some anti-diarrheal that will help with your digestion.

Cramps

Some people complain of cramps in the body. These can be muscle or other bodily cramps that might cause you to feel uncomfortable. So, it is important for you to restore the lost minerals from your body. The best way is to consume foods that are rich in the minerals. You can also consume more table salt. The cramps might not be limited to your muscles and might extend to your joints as well. Eat some fresh foods and nutrient oils to help with the process.

Kidney issues

This side effect is not that common but will mostly come about if you consume too much potassium. This can come through potassium supplements. It is important that you ask your physician if you can take the potassium supplement regularly. He will also prescribe the right amount that you have to take. Consuming a lot of water is a great way to deal with this issue.

Thyroid issues

Some people might also complain about thyroid issues, T3 to be precise. You will have to consult your physician and ask for a remedy that will help you move past it.

Lack of sleep

Some people complain of lack of sleep when on the ketogenic diet. This might be true owing to the imbalance on insulin and serotonin levels in the brain. The best solution is to increase the serotonin levels in your brain by taking up activities that will help you increase the serotonin levels such as exercising. Try also to avoid eating close to bedtime as that can cause you to lose sleep.

These are some of the common issues that come along with the ketogenic diet. there is no need for alarm. They will subside after a while as the body gets used to it. Instead of complaining about them, it is best to focus on the remedies to ease the symptoms.

Chapter 11: Related FAQs

Are ketogenic and other low carb diets the same?

The ketogenic diet is a diet that induces a state of ketosis. Ketosis refers to a situation where the body starts to burn away the fat and reduces the person's body weight. There are other diets such as the Atkin's diet, which is a low carb diet. But it might not provide the same benefits as the ketogenic diet. Both diets will provide different results and you can choose the one that suits your physique.

Is it bad to lose too much weight at once?

Generally, yes. You should try and lose weight slowly yet steadily. There must be progress with the weight loss. Do not try to lose all of it within a month or two. Have a weight loss plan in place that is practical. Try to lose not more than a few pounds a month. You should lose the weight based on your body type and weight. If you feel dizzy or weak then you should stop with the diet and consult with a physician to see if the problem can be fixed.

Can vegans take this diet up?

Yes. The low carb diet allows a wide range of foods to be consumed and does not limit it to just meats. You can consume fresh fruits and vegetables and also lentils. You can come up with a low carb vegan diet plan. If you don't know where to start, then you can research online and find an appropriate diet. Modify it as per your taste. The same extends to vegetarians who can make the addition of dairy products into their diet.

Is it important to consume lots of proteins as per the low carb diet?

Ideally yes. To make up for all the carbohydrates that are not consumed during the diet, it is important that you substitute it with the proteins. Proteins are known to help with weight reduction. It allows in the production of healthy muscles, which is great for the body. Most proteins come from foods that are part of our everyday diet. So all you have to do is increase their quantity and not go out of your way to incorporate it in your diet. Some of these include meats such as chicken, turkey, eggs, chickpeas, etc.

How much calories should I consume on a daily basis?

Calorie counting is often tricky. You have to know what each and every ingredient is in your meal and how many calories they carry. It can get a bit too tedious for you and you might give up on it altogether. However, it is best to have a rough idea of each meal and not get too serious about it. Calorie counting is a must no doubt but it is best if you have a rough estimate of how much you are consuming. Ideally, it is advisable to consume between 1500 and 1800 for women and between 1800 and 2200 for men. That will help you with your weight loss process as well.

Can I continue it for a lifetime?

Yes. It is a great idea for you to continue with the diet for a long time, possibly a lifetime. If you have the capacity to come up with timely meal plans that are easy to prepare then you will find it easy to settle in with the diet. You have to keep yourself motivated and keep aiming higher. There is nothing like being too fit and the more effort you put in, the better the results.

Are occasional drinks allowed?

Yes, occasional drinks are allowed provided they are low carb and not more than just a small glass. It is best to limit it to just a single drink per month and not any more. Speak with your family and friends. Tell them about your diet and that you will not be consuming any of the drinks that are prohibited as per the diet.

Are cheat meals allowed?

Yes. In fact, a cheat meal might be a must, as it will keep you motivated. You can use it as a reward and have it once in a while. The meal does not have to be a grand affair. It can be a simple burger or a pizza.

Chapter 12: Basic Exercise Plans

When it comes to your diet and exercise plan, it is important to follow a set sequence. Here are some of the exercises that you can take up.

Warm up

Warm up before taking up an exercise routine to avoid injuries. Warming up helps in preparing your body to take up the different exercises without feeling too tired. It is also important to not exercise with a cold body, as the heat will further help you burn fat. The warm up can be quite simple and yet very effective. The warm up routine may consist of a little running or jogging. If you wish to do something less, then you can jog on the spot or run on the treadmill for some time. You can also do something like stand and do a few jumping jacks. As long as your body heats up, it will work well for you.

Cardio exercises

Skipping

Skipping is a great activity that you can take up and quite easy as well. You can buy yourself a skipping rope and start skipping. Another way is to hold an imaginary skipping rope in your hand and start skipping. You can alternate between skipping and jumping jacks. Keep a count of your reps so that you don't over exercise or under exercise. You can also make use of a timer to keep time. How much you skip is up to you and you can choose the time or the count based on your capacity. Remember to do more first.

Jogging

Jogging is the next exercise that you can take up. Jogging is easy to take up and also quite effective. With jogging, all you have to do is find a walkway that is long enough and start taking small jumping steps. Don't mistake jogging with running, as the two are quite different. You can jog for around 30 minutes and then take a little rest. Start jogging again and then rest again. Such interval training will surely help your body feel a good burn. It is also best for all those that are unable to run.

Running

Running is great for anyone. In fact, you will see maximum weight loss when you run. It is best for you to pick morning time and start running early. You can do about 30 minutes to an hour. This will help with your weight loss. You can find a long walk way or can also run around in a circular motion. One good technique is to run for a minute and then jog for a minute. Run again and jog again. This will help your body get more in less time. Running is also ideal for those who wish to lose weight from their hip and lower abdomen. Running uphill will help with lower abdomen fat and running downhill helps with hip fat. You can run up and down a hill a few times.

Swimming

Swimming is not only easy to perform but also most effective when it comes to burning and eliminating fat from the body. You can hit the swimming pool 4 to 5 times a week and swim at least 20 laps. You can also do some running motion in the water as that will also help in weight loss. But you have to be serious about exercising and not simply pass your time at the pool.

Sports

Indulge in sports activities you like. Playing sports is quite fun. You can join your children or find a group you can play sports with. Sports activities get your heart rate up and will also help you feel relaxed. It can be anything like basketball or football or even baseball. As long as you run or jump around, your body will feel the burn. It is best for you to play sports at least 4 times a week.

Apart from these, you can engage in any other cardio exercise that you deem to be effective. It does not have to be picked from a particular list alone. If you think there is something else that will help you and your body, then do so.

Weight training

It might be important for you to weight train. Weight training involves lifting heavy weights. This is done to train your muscles and make your body more muscular. Weight training is pretty simple to undertake and it is important that you choose the right weights. For women, 5 lbs. is ideal while for men, its 10 lbs. You can increase the weights as you go. Some basic weight training exercises will suffice and you won't have to do too much. Just lifting your forearm up and down will do the trick. Try also the above the shoulder exercises as it will work on both the biceps and triceps. It is best to do weight training after some cardio, as that is when the body will feel the most burn. You can train with weights for 15 to 30 minutes or more if your body has the capacity for it.

Chin ups/ push ups

Chin-ups refer to holding a rod and pulling yourself up against your body weight. This will help you with your biceps and triceps. Hold your hands a little apart from each other. Lift yourself up and try to touch the rod using your chin. This is easier said than done and you should make use of the right technique to complete the motion. Push-ups are the opposite of chin-ups. You will have to place your palms on the floor in front of you. Now lift yourself up and lower your body down using just your arms. This is great for all those that wish to work on their obliques.

Resistance Crunches

Resistance crunches work much better than regular crunches, as they will cause you to put in a bit more effort. Here, you will place some weights on your abdomen or back when you perform the crunches. This will make it a bit difficult for you to perform the crunches. You can ask someone to place the weights on your body while you perform the crunches. Exercise a little precaution while performing the crunches to avoid any unnecessary injury.

Yoga/ tai chi

Yoga and tai chi poses are not body intensive yet will help in reducing your weight. Here are some poses that you can try.

Triangle pose

The triangle pose is quite easy to perform and great for your entire body. Start by standing straight with your hands by your side. Now spread your legs a little and bend down to your right side. Place your left palm next to your right foot and try not to bend your legs. Draw in a deep breath while bending down. Hold the pose for a couple of seconds and then raise your body up. Now bend to the other side. You can continue with this for the next 2 to 5 minutes.

Breathing exercises

Breathing exercises are great for you. Start by sitting on the floor and folding your legs. Now, draw in deep breaths. Focus on your breath and ensure that your exhaled breath is slightly more paced as compared to your inhaled breath. You should literally feel your lower stomach move in and out. Alternately, you can try out Anulom Vilom where you alternate your nostrils to draw in and exhale breath. Both will help you reduce the fat in your stomach or at least loosen it to some extent.

Bridge pose

The bridge pose is for your back muscles. Start by lying on your back. Now bend your knees such that they point to the sky. Use your palms to bring your heels close to your butt. Now raise your lower back and support your upper body with your shoulders. You can place your hands under your back and interlock your fingers. Hold the pose for a while and then lower yourself down. Repeat the same again.

Tree pose

Tree pose is easy to perform. Stand straight with your hands by your side. Then lift your feet up using your hands and place it on the inner side of your thigh. Maintain your balance and lift your hands up in the air to make a Namaste above your head. Hold the pose for a few seconds and then lower your hands back down. Now repeat it with the other foot.

Bow pose

Bow pose helps with abs and lower back fat. Lie flat on the ground. Lift up your upper body and also your lower body simultaneously. Now hold your ankles using your palms and pull them in towards your butt. You should push your head as back as possible while looking upwards. Maintain the pose for a few seconds and go back to neutral. Assume the same pose again, wait and release. Keep doing this for the next 5 to 10 minutes.

You don't have to always be too rigorous to lose weight. You can make use of a set of simple movement based exercises as well. Take advantage of the Internet to look up more tai chi poses that you can do. These are just a few of the different exercises you can incorporate in your work out plan to remain fit and healthy.

Chapter 13: Precautions to Observe on the Diet

There are a few precautions that you have to observe when it comes to the ketogenic diet. Here they are:

Pregnant women

The diet is safe for most people and might also include pregnant women. Still, consulting your doctor first is the best move to do. He might prescribe a diet that will settle in with you and your unborn baby. The keto diet side effects might aggravate the hormonal imbalances and bodily changes during pregnancy and put a stress on the body more. It is best to wait after you had your baby and had settled to the life changes that comes with it before taking on the keto diet. If you have been on the diet while getting pregnant then you might not need to make too many modifications to it. Still, consulting your doctor is a must.

Post delivery

New mothers have to consult a doctor as the body needs some time to recover. It is best not to rush into it. Also, the doctor might suggest something else to help you get back to your pre-pregnancy body and still remain fit.

Elders

It is important for elders to consult a doctor as well and know if any modifications are needed to be made in the diet. Get a list of supplements and other things that will help with the diet. The doctor might also modify some of the medications being taken.

Children

Parents need to exercise a little precaution when it comes to putting their children on the ketogenic diet. Because of their age and special nutritional needs, their diets might have to be modified a bit. You can work closely with a dietician to come up with a diet plan. If your child is quite fat, plan an exercise routine along with the diet plan to help avail dual benefits.

Illness

If you already suffer from a condition like diabetes or heart disease, speak with your doctor beforehand for appropriate advice. If you are taking any medications, then you can ask if you can take the medicine along with the diet.

Supplements

Before you take any of the supplements, it is best that you ask your doctor first. He will tell you if it is safe to consume them. Some supplements might also react with some medicines and so you will have to ask your physician. The dosages will also differ from person to person thus be careful with the dosage.

These are some of the cases where extra precautions are needed. Somehow, they should not deter you from taking up the diet.

Chapter 14: How to Stick to The Low Carb Diet

When it comes to taking up a new diet, it is obvious that both your body and mind will resist it. Certain measures are needed to make the habit stay. This chapter will look on the steps on how to stick to your diet.

Do your research

The first and foremost advice is to do as much research on the topic as possible. Research will help you know what the diet is and how you can go about it. This book will give you a lot of information on the diet and how to go about it no doubt. Still, do not limit yourself to just the information present in this book. It is important that you look outside it as well. You will have to look for websites that will give you valuable and reliable information on the topic and also increase its worth. You can also turn to some publications for the same. A little research and understanding will go a long way towards helping you turn it into a lifetime habit.

Create a time table

A timetable will come in handy and help you carry out your diet easily. The timetable can be simple with the different activities and the respective timings mentioned next to it. You can make two columns where the first one mentions the activity and the other column the time. The activities can be like eat a snack, exercise etc.

Anything that helps you stick with the diet will cause you to remain with it for a long time.

Maintain a record

Many people find it extremely motivating to maintain a record of their experiences. They prefer to maintain a journal and write down their daily experiences with the diet. This can include the effects that the diet have on the body, weight loss, higher energy levels, etc. You will see your progress better and that your body is getting fitter. It will motivate you to continue with the diet for long and not stop with it. You can either maintain a physical journal or a digital one. A digital one will be easy to maintain and also refer back.

Find a partner

A partner will not only help you remain motivated to continue with the diet but also make it easier for you. You will not have to prepare different meals for the different members of your family. If all of them are following the diet with you, then the meals will be quite easy to prepare. If your spouse is also following the diet, then he or she might help you stay on course. But it need not always be a spouse, a friend or a sibling can be your partner as well.

Find a group

Just like a partner, you can also choose to join a group. The group can be a ketogenic diet group that meets up in your area to discuss the effects of the diet and also other aspects of it. If the group is not present in your area, then you can create one yourself. Just ask your friends if they are interested in it or already follow the diet. Then invite them over and discuss the diet in detail with them. That will surely help you remain with the diet for long.

Prepare meal plans

Meal plans are a great way to feel motivated to follow the ketogenic diet. You can create the meal plans well in advance and follow them through. We've included some basic meal plans that you can follow and also some recipes that you can try out. These will surely give you a head start. You can also consider cleaning up your kitchen by disposing off the fatty and sugary foods and stacking up on the healthy and keto friendly foods. This will help you remain motivated.

Appreciate your body

Those who love their body and remain appreciative of it will find it rather easy to maintain a diet. They will not take it for granted and put in necessary efforts to maintain a slim and trim body. The same will extend to you if you wish to make full use of the ketogenic diet. You have to appreciate your body to keep it healthy. Take some time out to go through your diet once in a while and see if it is helping you remain fit and healthy.

Reward yourself

Nothing works better than rewarding yourself with something nice from time to time. This need not be a food reward. Although many people would consider the celebration meal to be a reward in itself, you might have to do much more. This can include visiting a spa for a relaxing massage, taking a vacation, buying yourself something nice, etc. All of it will go a long way in helping you remain in the diet. But make sure you don't reward yourself too often and to leave a little gap between one reward and the next.

Speak about it

It is a good idea for you to speak about the diet to as many people as possible. You can also profess about it as that will motivate your further. You can try speaking about it on an online site or blog about it. You can also post pictures of yourself from before and after. That will help you remain motivated and continue with the diet for a long time. However, you must prepare to read a few nasty comments about the diet. They might seem harsh. Learn to ignore them and focus on the positive ones.

These are just some of the things that you can do to remain motivated with the diet. Do not be limited to just these. Be creative and do whatever it takes to stick with your diet.

Chapter 15: Sumptuous Recipes

Breakfast recipes

Cheddar omelet with fresh salad

Ingredients:
- 3 large eggs, slightly beaten
- 1 tablespoon mixed herbs, parsley, basil, cilantro, chopped
- Salt to taste
- Black pepper to taste
- 1 tablespoon unsalted butter
- 2 tablespoons fresh goat cheese

Recipe:

Place the griddle on heat. Combine the eggs, herbs (reserve some for the cheese), salt and pepper in a bowl and whisk until well combined. Add the butter to the pan and allow it to melt. Put the beaten eggs to make an omelet. While the egg is cooking, place the cheese in a bowl and crumble it along with the herbs and mix well. Open the omelet on a plate and sprinkle the goat's cheese. Fold the omelet and serve hot.

Chicken and mushroom breakfast

Ingredients:
- 4 small eggs
- 2 chicken Breast, skinned
- 3 tablespoons scallions, chopped

- 2 tablespoons Olive Oil
- 1 cup mushrooms, chopped
- Salt to taste
- Black pepper to taste
- Italian seasoning, to taste
- 1/4 cup shredded Mozzarella Cheese

Recipe:

Beat the eggs in a bowl along with the salt, pepper and seasoning and mix until well combined. Cut the chicken breasts into small pieces and add it to the egg mix. Meanwhile, add the oil to the pan and allow it to heat. Sauté the chopped scallions. Add in the mushrooms and the marinated chicken. Sauté until the chicken is soft. Remove from pan, sprinkle the mozzarella on top and serve hot.

Lunch recipes

Stuffed bottle gourd

Ingredients:
- 1 large bottle gourd
- 1 large red onion, chopped
- 1 large tomato, chopped
- 2 tablespoons garlic
- ½ inch ginger stick, peeled and grated
- 1 tablespoon oil
- Salt to taste
- Pepper to taste
- ¼ the cup mozzarella cheese

Recipe:

Heat oil and sauté chopped onions and garlic in a pan. Once it browns, add in the tomato, salt and pepper. Give it a good mix. Meanwhile, preheat the oven to 350 degrees Fahrenheit. Cut the top of the bottle gourd and cut it into 3 to 4 cylinders. Use a spoon to scoop out the centers of the gourd and add it to the tomato mix. Place the cylinders on a baking tray. Fill each of them with the tomato mix and sprinkle the cheese on top.

Place it in the oven for 20 to 30 minutes. Serve hot.

Chickpea salad

Ingredients:
- 1 cup chickpeas, boiled
- 1 large tomato
- 1 red onion
- 1 zucchini
- 1 tablespoon olive oil
- 1 tablespoon mustard
- Salt to taste
- Pepper to taste

Recipe:

Chop the tomatoes, onion and zucchini into small pieces. Add the mustard and oil to a small bowl and mix until well combined. Add the chickpeas to a bowl along with the chopped vegetables. Now add the salt and pepper and mix until well combined.

Add in the mustard and oil paste and serve.

Dinner recipes

Shrimpy devilled eggs

Ingredients:
- 4 large Boiled Eggs
- 2 tablespoons low fat mayonnaise, homemade or store bought

- 2 tablespoons pickles
- 1/2 teaspoon mustard
- 1/2 teaspoon horseradish (optional)
- 1/8 teaspoon pepper sauce
- 8 fresh larges shrimps
- Salt to taste
- Cilantro to sprinkle

Recipe:

Cut the eggs into half and scoop out the yellow from the center. Put it in a bowl along with the mayonnaise, pickle, horseradish, mustard, pepper sauce and salt. Mix well. Now spoon a teaspoon or so of the yolk mix inside the egg halves. Place one shrimp each on top of each of the yolk. You can press it in a little to help it stay in place. Sprinkle some of the cilantro on top and serve.

Turkey sausages

Ingredients:
- 2 tablespoons onions, chopped
- 1 cup turkey Sausages, cut into pieces
- 1 tablespoon oil
- Salt to taste
- Pepper to taste
- 1/3 cup chopped green pepper
- 2 tablespoons mozzarella cheese

Recipe:

Heat the oil in a pan. Add in the chopped onion. Allow it to sauté for a while or until it browns. Then add in the green pepper along with the salt and pepper and give it a good mix. Add in the sausages and sauté it until it browns and softens. Sprinkle the cheese on top and serve hot.

Ketogenic drink recipes

Simple lemon tea

Ingredients:
- 1 teaspoon regular tea powder
- 1 lemon
- 1 cup water
- ½ teaspoon honey, optional

Recipe:
Heat water in a pan. Add the tea powder and allow it to boil. Then strain it into a cup. Squeeze in the lemon and mix well. Add in the honey, stir and serve hot. This can also be cooled and served as cold tea.

Cleansing drink

Ingredients:
- 1 cup kale, chopped
- ½ cup green peppers, chopped
- 1 zucchini
- Salt
- Coconut milk as needed

Recipe:
Add all the ingredients to a blender and make a smooth puree. Add in as much coconut milk as needed and serve.

Easy juice pops

Ingredients:
- 1 cup melon pieces
- 1 cup papaya pieces
- 1 cup strawberries

- 1 cup blueberries
- ½ cup lemon juice
- ½ cup fresh mint leaves, chopped

Recipe:

Put all the fruits in a juicer and make a fresh juice. Add in the lemon juice and mix well. Pour the juice into Popsicle molds. Drop in a few mint leaves into each and freeze.

Black tea infuse

Ingredients:
- 2 black tea bags
- 2 cups water
- 1 cup rose petals
- Honey to taste (optional)

Recipe:

Boil water in a pan. Add in the rose petals and allow it to infuse. Put the tea bags in a cup. Add in the rose infused water and allow the tea bag to steep for a while. Serve it hot.

Green tea with fruits

Ingredients:
- 2 green tea bags
- 2 cups water
- ½ cup apples, chopped
- ½ cup grapes, whole
- ½ cup melon, chopped
- Hone to taste

Recipe:

Boil water in a pan. Put the tea bags in a cup and pour the hot water. Put cut fruits in a bowl and add the honey. Mix well. Pour the tea on top and mix. Serve cold.

Coconut surprise

Ingredients:
- 1 cup coconut water
- ½ cup coconut cream
- ½ cup pineapple, chopped
- Honey to taste
- Mint leaves to sprinkle.

Recipe:
Put the coconut cream and pineapple pieces in a blender and whizz until smooth. Add the honey and coconut water and whizz again until well blended. Add in some crushed ice to the mix. Serve cold with a few mint leaves sprinkled on top.

Chapter 16: Shopping List to Carry with you / 1 Week Ketogenic Diet Plan

Aisles to avoid

- Processed, refined sugars: soft drinks, store bought juices, agave, candies, ice creams and other processed foods that contain sugar.
- Gluten Grains: Wheat, oats, rye, barley and all foods made from these.
- Trans Fats: Anything marked as hydrogenated or poly hydrogenated.
- High-level Omega-6 oils and Vegetable Oils: sunflower, safflower, pomace, cottonseed oil, soya bean oil, etc.
- Artificial Sweeteners: None of the ready available brands are allowed for consumption. Sauces and condiments.
- Any products that carry diet or low fat markings. They all might contain unnecessary chemicals.
- Any other processed foods that you think are not right for you or your diet. Avoid consuming any unnecessary readymade foods.
-

Shopping list to carry with you

- Meat: chicken, lamb, beef, pork and other grass fed meat
- Fish: bass, trout, salmon and other wild fish
- Eggs: Free-range eggs

- Vegetables: Broccoli, Spinach, carrots, cauliflower, and many others
- Fruits: kiwis, pineapples, apples, papaya, watermelon, blueberries, strawberries, etc.
- Nuts - Seeds: walnuts, pine nuts, hazel nuts, cashew nuts, and almonds
- High-Fat Dairy: yogurt, cheese, cream, butter, ghee
- Fats and Oils: olive oil, coconut oil, almond oil, cashew oil, and groundnut oil
-

Monday

Breakfast: Omelet with goat's cheese (recipe included in this book)
Lunch: Low fat fresh yogurt with strawberries and a few cashews roasted and slivered (make sure the fat from it does not escape while roasting)
Dinner: simple vegetable salad dressed with cold fresh low fat yogurt

Tuesday

Breakfast: chicken and mushroom breakfast (recipe included in this book)
Lunch: Any leftover fresh vegetable salad with cold fresh yogurt, you can add in some fresh vegetables if you like.
Dinner: sautéed vegetables with grilled chicken and hot sauce

Wednesday

Breakfast: egg frittata with colorful vegetables
Lunch: baked salmon with some olive oil and garlic drizzle
Dinner: fruit salad with a little strawberry yogurt

Thursday

Breakfast: left over fruit salad with strawberry yogurt, add in some fresh fruits to it
Lunch: cleansing smoothie with kale, pepper, MCT oil and cucumbers
Dinner: chicken patties with roasted vegetables

Friday

Breakfast: omelets with crispy bacon
Lunch: shrimp cocktail with low fat yogurt sauce
Dinner: beef stew

Saturday

Breakfast: devilled eggs with avocado
Lunch: pork ribs roasted and salsa sauce
Dinner: mixed vegetable salad with fresh yogurt

Sunday

Breakfast: left over mixed vegetable salad with fresh yogurt, add in some fresh vegetables
Lunch: spicy chicken breasts with cauliflower rice
Dinner: one cheat meal, 1 small burger with ideally whole-wheat bun

This is a good meal plan to start with to help you get started with the diet at the earliest.

Chapter 17: Things You Will Need While On the Diet

When it comes to losing weight and body fat, it is best that you do everything in your power to see results. In this chapter, we will look at some of the things that you may need to continue with the diet for a long time.

Weighing machine

You have to buy yourself a weighing machine. It is probably the most important thing that you will need for your journey. Many people argue that a person's weight does not really tell whether he or she is fat. There is water weight and also bone density to account for. However, it will give an accurate measure of your real weight. It will tell you how heavy you really are and how much weight you should have. You can either buy a digital one or a conventional machine. The former will give you an accurate measure.

Pressure cooker

Buying a pressure cooker for yourself will prove to be a big boon. You will find it quite easy to cook your meals without having to put in too much effort. All you do is put in all the ingredients, add water and allow it to blow 3 to 5 whistles. Wait for the steam to escape and your meal will be ready. It will be a one-pot solution that will surely help you cook the meals fast.

Instant pot

You can also buy yourself an instant pot. It is a pressure cooker, a slow cooker and a steamer all in one. This generally run on electricity and will help you cook with ease. It also have an instant steam release vent that will help release the steam fast. It is also good to reheat food. A slow cooker will help you cook the food slowly and help preserve most of the nutrition in the food. All you have to do is put the food into the instant pot and the food will be hot and ready in no time at all.

Body fat machine

A body fat machine is different from a weighing machine. It is one that will help measure the fat in your body. A person might appear slim but the fat content in the body might be more. So, you will have to buy a body fat percentage monitor to see how much fat is present in your body. The limit differs from person to person but in general it is limited to 6% per person. You can know the exact values by doing a quick Internet search.

Tea infuser

We looked at some easy tea recipes that you can try out. They will help you beat your hunger pangs and also cleanse your body from the inside. You can buy a tea infuser to help you prepare the tea with ease. All you have to do is add in some powder or leaves in one section and some hot water in the other and your tea will be infused. You don't have to worry about heating water or finding a strainer. You can simply strain the tea into a cup with much ease.

Air fryer

The latest technology in the world of health care is an air fryer. The air fryer is one where you will not need to use too much oil to prepare food. You will only have to apply a little by making use of a brush. You won't have to bust out the deep fryer and your fritters and other such food items will be ready within no time. This is great for people looking to eat their favorite foods without the added carbs or calories.

Miscellaneous

Apart from these, you can also buy some other things that you think will help you with your weight loss journey. You can buy a few ketogenic recipe books if you like or also a ketogenic food chart. These will help you stay on course.

Key highlights

First and foremost, it is important to understand what the ketogenic diet is all about. If you don't know what it means or stands for and simply decide to take it up, then it will not work for you. Put in efforts to do as much research on the topic as possible.

As you know by now, the keto diet is a low carb diet. Low carb refers to low carbohydrates that are to be consumed by the dieter. Carbohydrates give people the sugar or energy to survive. But too much of it will cause it to be converted to fat. So, by consuming less carbohydrates and increasing the protein intake, you will successfully burn the fat in the body. Therefore, these diets are great for all those that wish to attain a slim body.

The next thing is to plan out your diet. It is important to have a set plan. Do not randomly start on it and expect to see results. Have a schedule in place. Start by weighing yourself and then deciding on how much you plan to lose. Based on it you can come up with the ketogenic plan. The main aim of the plan is to cut down on the consumption of carbohydrates. Schedule it either for more than a week or a month. It is important to plan it out in a way that you can stick with it from start to finish. Be inspired by other people who have taken up the diet. You can try asking them and coming up with a plan for yourself. But don't copy the plan as is. It should cater to your body type and must not be generic in nature. The plan should be such that it helps you with your weight loss mission and is not a fancy timetable for you.

There are some mistakes to watch out for when you are on the diet. These mistakes might cause you to go back to your old eating patterns and habits and might reduce its effectivity on your body.

The ketogenic diet comes with a few common side effects. They are a part and parcel of the diet and you will experience some or all of them at some point during your diet. However, precautionary measures are available to counter them. Once your body gets used to the diet, you will not feel like they are big problems at all. Learn to look past them and remain focused on your diet.

We've given some of the best recipes you can try. These recipes are all easy to prepare and will not take too much time. Ensure all the ingredients are ready before hand so that you can reach into the right boxes and cook them for mealtimes. You can also make them in advance and keep them in the fridge. Grab and go meals will surely help you remain fit and healthy.

Some cleaning up will be necessary to stay on course like clearing out your current kitchen or pantry and throwing out all the unnecessary foods, stacking up on foods that are in keeping with the diet, etc. These will help you remain motivated and will do more towards turning it into a habit. Bring a shopping list with all the different foods that are allowed in the diet when you hit the supermarket. You can also buy them online and order from the same list on a monthly basis.

The meal plans that were mentioned in this book are meant to help you get a head start. You can either make use of the same or use it as a blueprint to come up with your own meal plans. They will surely help you prepare the meals with ease and not have to sweat it out. Encourage your family members to take up the diet with you and avail its benefits. It will also be easy for you, as you will only have to prepare one meal and not different ones.

The diet is great for weight loss no doubt but you will have to consume a few supplements in order to help your body remain fit and healthy. Consult with your physician to know which supplements will suit your body. This step is especially important if you are pregnant or nursing or are a senior citizen. These supplements might also react with some medicines that you are already taking and so, it is best that you consult your physician first. Most of these supplements are available over the counter but you might need a prescription for others.

It is extremely important for you to exercise in order to lose weight faster. A healthy diet will not suffice, especially if you plan on losing weight at an elevated pace. Come up with an exercise plan that will help in burning the fat and also get the body to burn away the sugar and carbohydrates. Those who do not exercise and rely only on the diet might see slower results and in some cases, the lost weight is added back on.

There are many things that you can do to stay on the diet. Try and do your best to convert the ketogenic diet into a lifetime choice. Some of the ideas include rewarding yourself, joining a group etc. Do whatever you think will work for you best to stay on course. Once you start seeing the results, you will be motivated to stick with the diet and reel in both health and happiness.

Conclusion

Thank you once again for choosing this book.

Ketogenic diet is a way of life and all about improving your health by working along with your body and not against it. Experiment with the diet and exercise options available, keep track of your progress and find which works best for you.

Get started right now. It is not that difficult, a little bit of effort can work wonders for you! So get going and all the best!

Thank you!

Lean Diet:

6 Weeks To Becoming A Lean Green Eating Machine!

The following information is presented purely for informative purposes and is therefore considered universal. The information presented within is done so without a contract or any other type of assurance as to its quality or validity.

Any trademarks which are used are done so without consent and any use of the same does not imply consent or permission was gained from the owner. Any trademarks or brands found within are purely used for clarification purposes and no owners are in anyway affiliated with this work.

Introduction

Making a major dietary change isn't easy and choosing this book or others like it is a great first step. Inside you will learn everything there is to know about the lean diet and how it can help you lose weight and build muscle mass at the same time.

This book contains proven steps and strategies designed to ensure you make the most out of your dieting experience in one of the healthiest, and least restrictive diets around. That doesn't mean it is for everyone, however, which is why it is important to always consult a dietitian or healthcare professional before making any major dietary changes. This is always recommended to ensure you aren't accidentally doing yourself more harm than good. With that in mind, get ready to start on the road to a healthier and happier you!

Thanks again for downloading this book, I hope you enjoy it!

Chapter 1: All About the Lean Diet

Unlike many diet plans that are all about skewing your diet towards one extreme or another or counting the caloric content of every single thing you eat, the Lean diet is all about moderation. A good lean meal is part protein, part healthy carbohydrates and part healthy fats; and more importantly, it is low in processed ingredients or excessive sugar. The only thing you need to worry about is how natural an individual piece of food is, the rest takes care of itself.

Foods that are encouraged on the lean diet are those that are broadly considered clean, that is, those that are not processed which means they are free of chemical colorings, flavorings or textures, preservatives and additives. As a general rule, the higher the percentage of processed ingredients something has, the less nutrition it actually has as well. Your goal should be to moderate your carbohydrate intake to reasonable levels and decrease your sugar intake drastically as well. Outside of the general food restrictions, the lean diet can be broken down into several main principles.

Account for what you eat

Aside from eating as many naturally occurring foods as possible, the other biggest thing to consider when striving to follow a lean lifestyle is that, while not actively counting calories, you do need to be aware of what is going into and being burned up by your body. This is determined by your metabolism which is a combination of how you digest food, which accounts for roughly 10 percent of your total metabolism. You can improve your general digestion rate by eating more protein as a greater portion of protein calories are burned while swallowing as opposed to other types of food.

It is likewise important to make a conscious effort to get up and move more, as the amount you move is directly related to roughly 30 percent of your total metabolism. This is one of the reasons it is so important to exercise regularly when following the lean diet as discussed in chapter 2. The rest of your metabolism is committed to automated bodily functions which is why simply cutting your caloric intake indiscriminately never really works. Instead, this simply leaves you with less energy overall which slows your metabolism and makes it more likely for your body to hang on to every calorie.

When it comes to eating regularly, your thoughts are also going to have to change. When following a lean lifestyle, you should plan on eating 3 regular sized meals as well as two protein rich snacks each and every day. This will help your metabolism stay at a more consistent rate by preventing both blood sugar and insulin levels from spiking and crashing as it common with the standard 3 meal cycle. When it comes to portion sizes, you should limit proteins to those the size of your open hand and carbohydrates to the size of a first. Eat as many healthy vegetables as you like.

Find better fuel

Following a lean lifestyle means that some 80 percent of the food you each should have no ingredient labels. This means things like beans, potatoes, vegetables, fruits, seeds, nuts, milk, eggs, fish and grass-fed animals. 10 percent should be devoted strictly to the additional protein that you will need in order to make the most of the lean diet (1 gram per pound of body weight) this generally means protein powders which are fine as long as they contain very little sugar. The remaining 10 percent should also be made up of foods that you don't eat regularly, to expand your nutrient portfolio as well as your horizons.

Know your targets

To follow the lean diet successfully, you will need to consume protein for approximately 30 percent of your total daily intake. Protein is beneficial for losing weight because it makes you feel full longer, while also improving your metabolism and maintaining your muscle mass. Depending on the amount of weight you are interested in losing, you will want to aim for between .5 and .7 grams of fat per pound of body weight. The more you have to lose, the greater the amount of fat per pound you will want to start with.

These fats should all be of the healthy variety which includes things like palm oil, avocados, eggs, lard, chicken fat, coconut oil, clarified butter, ghee and beef tallow. Fats to avoid include canola oil, blended oils, saturated fats and most salad dressing. A higher percentage of healthy fat in your diet will mean a decrease in the overall number of carbohydrates you consume which means your body will burn fat for energy instead.

Do the math

With these numbers in mind, all you have to do is plug in your own specifics and figure out the details that are right for you. From there, all you need to do is figure out how many calories you are burning as you exercise and make a point of consuming a smaller amount each day than what you expend. Once you have a series of concrete goals in mind you will find that it is much easier to get started as there are clear metrics for success and failure in place.

The meal plan outlined in chapters 4 through 9 was designed with a 165 lbs. individual in mind who is following the exercise guide outlined in chapter 2. Make sure to alter it to fit your specifics with that in mind. Consider the recipes outlined within as a guidebook to indicate the sorts of meals you should be looking for when it comes to planning out the meal plan that works for you.

Chapter 2: Exercise and the Lean Diet

One of the best benefits of the lean diet is that, in addition to being extremely healthy, it naturally puts the body in a state that makes it easier to shed fat and build muscle. It is important to build on these natural proclivities by committing to an exercise program similar to the one outlined below.

The following exercise plan is for those who are already at a moderate to good level of fitness. If you aren't quite there yet, simply choose a few exercises from the list each day and add additional exercises as you feel you are able. Remember, it is important to choose weights that allow you to complete the number of sets and repetitions listed with only a moderate amount of struggle.

If the exercises are too easy, increase the weight being used, if they are too hard, go down a weight instead. It is important to always use the right weights for you, if you go too light on the weight then you are simply wasting time, commit to exercising regularly or you are cheating yourself out of the true efficacy of the lean diet. Don't forget to warm up for approximately 10 minutes before starting your training for the day and don't underestimate the benefits of a cool down period as well.

Week 1 Day 1 Biceps and Back

- *Bent over twin dumbbell row:* Do 2 sets of between 10 and 12 repetitions if you can, do at least 1 set if possible.

- *Pullups:* Do 2 sets of between 10 and 12 repetitions if you can, do at least 1 set if possible.

- *Standing Wide Grip Barbell Curl:* Do 2 sets of between 10 and 12 repetitions if you can, do at least 1 set if possible.

- *Alternating Dumbbell Bicep Curl:* Do 2 sets of between 10 and 12 repetitions if you can, do at least 1 set if possible.

- *Elliptical:* 1 or 2 minutes on an easy resistance, between 1 and 3 minutes on a moderate resistance, between 1 and 3 minutes on a difficult resistance, alternate between resistance level 2 and resistance level 3 for between 8 and 10 minutes, between 1 and 3 minutes on medium resistance and between 1 and 2 minutes on easy resistance. Shoot for between 25 and 30 minutes' total.

Tips

- It is important to always use the correct form to make sure you get the most effective, and safest workout possible.

- Ideally, you want each repetition to take about 2 seconds to complete the lift portion and no more than 3 seconds to return to the original position.

- Never swing the weights, always remain complete control. This means not letting gravity do the work on the return to the starting positon.

- Rest as long as you need to catch your breath, don't milk it, however, and work to maintain a steady heart rate.

Week 1 Day 2 Triceps, Shoulders, Chest

- *Medium Grip Barbell Bench Press:* Do 2 sets of between 10 and 12 repetitions if you can, do at least 1 set if possible.

- *Twisting Dumbbell Fly Inclines*: Do 2 sets of between 10 and 12 repetitions if you can, do at least 1 set if possible.

- *Sitting Dumbbell Press:* Do 2 sets of between 10 and 12 repetitions if you can, do at least 1 set if possible.

- *Lateral Side Raises:* Do 2 sets of between 10 and 12 repetitions if you can, do at least 1 set if possible.

- *Overhead Triceps Press:* Do 2 sets of between 10 and 12 repetitions if you can, do at least 1 set if possible.

- *Dips:* Do 2 sets of between 10 and 12 repetitions if you can, do at least 1 set if possible.

Tips

- When warming up, it is important to get your tendons and muscles heated up and elastic enough for the trials ahead. Always warm up and cool down to help prevent injury.

- When lifting your goal should be to simulate your muscles, not to annihilate them. Lifting an overly heavy weight will actually break down your muscles, not help them get stronger. Lift the right amount and you will see steadier progress over time.

- When it comes to resting, try and rest a minute or less between arms or abs sets and no more than 2 minutes between leg sets for the best results.

Week 1 Day 3 Cardio Only

- *Elliptical:* 1 or 2 minutes on an easy resistance, between 1 and 3 minutes on a moderate resistance, between 1 and 3 minutes on a difficult resistance, alternate between resistance level 2 and resistance level 3 for between 8 and 10 minutes, between 1 and 3 minutes on medium resistance and between 1 and 2 minutes on easy resistance. Shoot for between 25 and 30 minutes' total.

Week 1 Day 4 Abs and Legs

- *Barbell Squats:* Do 2 sets of between 10 and 12 repetitions if you can, do at least 1 set if possible.

- *Lunges with Dumbbells:* Do 2 sets of between 10 and 12 repetitions if you can, do at least 1 set if possible.

- *Reverse Leg Curls:* Do 2 sets of between 10 and 12 repetitions if you can, do at least 1 set if possible.

- *Stiff Leg Deadlift Barbell:* Do 2 sets of between 10 and 12 repetitions if you can, do at least 1 set if possible.

- *Sitting Calf Raise:* Do 2 sets of between 10 and 12 repetitions if you can, do at least 1 set if possible.

- *Calf Raises Standing:* Do 2 sets of between 10 and 12 repetitions if you can, do at least 1 set if possible.

- *Crunches:* Do 2 sets of between 10 and 12 repetitions if you can, do at least 1 set if possible.

You are likely going to be feeling a bit sore after hitting the legs so hard today so it is extremely important that you stretch after you have finished working out. Do yourself a favor and plan for a little extra sleep tonight as well.

Week 1 Day 5 Biceps and Back

- *Pullups:* Do 2 sets of between 10 and 12 repetitions if you can, do at least 1 set if possible.

- *Dumbbell Rows:* Do 2 sets of between 10 and 12 repetitions if you can, do at least 1 set if possible.

- *Back Extensions:* Do 2 sets of between 10 and 12 repetitions if you can, do at least 1 set if possible.

- *Concentration curls:* Do 2 sets of between 10 and 12 repetitions if you can, do at least 1 set if possible.

- *Preacher Curls:* Do 2 sets of between 10 and 12 repetitions if you can, do at least 1 set if possible.

- *Elliptical:* 1 or 2 minutes on an easy resistance, between 1 and 3 minutes on a moderate resistance, between 1 and 3 minutes on a difficult resistance, alternate between resistance level 2 and resistance level 3 for between 8 and 10 minutes, between 1 and 3 minutes on medium resistance and between 1 and 2 minutes on easy resistance. Shoot for between 25 and 30 minutes' total.

Week 1, Day 6 Cardio

- *Elliptical:* 1 or 2 minutes on an easy resistance, between 1 and 3 minutes on a moderate resistance, between 1 and 3 minutes on a difficult resistance, alternate between resistance level 2 and resistance level 3 for between 8 and 10 minutes, between 1 and 3 minutes on medium resistance and between 1 and 2 minutes on easy resistance. Shoot for between 25 and 30 minutes' total.

Week 1, Day 7 Triceps, Shoulders, Chest

- *Medium Grip Incline Barbell Bench Press:* Do 2 sets of between 10 and 12 repetitions if you can, do at least 1 set if possible.

- *Butterfly:* Do 2 sets of between 10 and 12 repetitions if you can, do at least 1 set if possible.

- *Lateral Side raise:* Do 2 sets of between 10 and 12 repetitions if you can, do at least 1 set if possible.

- *Sitting Dumbbell Press:* Do 2 sets of between 10 and 12 repetitions if you can, do at least 1 set if possible.

- *Pushdown for Triceps:* Do 2 sets of between 10 and 12 repetitions if you can, do at least 1 set if possible.

- *Overhead Barbell Triceps Extensions:* Do 2 sets of between 10 and 12 repetitions if you can, do at least 1 set if possible.

Week 2, Day 1 Abs and Legs

- *Leg Press:* Do 2 sets of between 10 and 12 repetitions if you can, do at least 1 set if possible.

- *Leg Extensions:* Do 2 sets of between 10 and 12 repetitions if you can, do at least 1 set if possible.

- *Sitting Leg Curl:* Do 2 sets of between 10 and 12 repetitions if you can, do at least 1 set if possible.

- *Dumbbell Deadlift:* Do 2 sets of between 10 and 12 repetitions if you can, do at least 1 set if possible.

- *Sitting Calf Raise:* Do 2 sets of between 10 and 12 repetitions if you can, do at least 1 set if possible.

- *Crunches:* Do 2 sets of between 10 and 12 repetitions if you can, do at least 1 set if possible.

- *Hanging Leg Raise:* Do 2 sets of between 10 and 12 repetitions if you can, do at least 1 set if possible.

Week 2, Day 2 Cardio

- *Elliptical:* 1 or 2 minutes on an easy resistance, between 1 and 3 minutes on a moderate resistance, between 1 and 3 minutes on a difficult resistance, alternate between resistance level 2 and resistance level 3 for between 8 and 10 minutes, between 1 and 3 minutes on medium resistance and between 1 and 2 minutes on easy resistance. Shoot for between 25 and 30 minutes' total.

Week 2, Day 3 Biceps and Back

- *Single Arm Dumbbell Rows:* Do 2 sets of between 10 and 12 repetitions if you can, do at least 1 set if possible.

- *Cable Pulldowns:* Do 2 sets of between 10 and 12 repetitions if you can, do at least 1 set if possible.

- *Barbell Deadlifts:* Do 2 sets of between 10 and 12 repetitions if you can, do at least 1 set if possible.

- *Alternating Bicep Curls:* Do 2 sets of between 10 and 12 repetitions if you can, do at least 1 set if possible.

- *Standing Cable Curls:* Do 2 sets of between 10 and 12 repetitions if you can, do at least 1 set if possible.

- *Elliptical:* 1 or 2 minutes on an easy resistance, between 1 and 3 minutes on a moderate resistance, between 1 and 3 minutes on a difficult resistance, alternate between resistance level 2 and resistance level 3 for between 8 and 10 minutes, between 1 and 3 minutes on medium resistance and between 1 and 2 minutes on easy resistance. Shoot for between 25 and 30 minutes' total.

Week 2, Day 4 Shoulders, Triceps and Chest

- *Medium Grip Barbell Bench Press:* Do 2 sets of between 10 and 12 repetitions if you can, do at least 1 set if possible.

- *Dumbbell Flies (Inclined):* Do 2 sets of between 10 and 12 repetitions if you can, do at least 1 set if possible.

- *Seated Rear Deltoid Muscle Raise:* Do 2 sets of between 10 and 12 repetitions if you can, do at least 1 set if possible.

- *Triceps Dips:* Do 2 sets of between 10 and 12 repetitions if you can, do at least 1 set if possible.

Week 2, Day 5 Cardio

- *Elliptical:* 1 or 2 minutes on an easy resistance, between 1 and 3 minutes on a moderate resistance, between 1 and 3 minutes on a difficult resistance, alternate between resistance level 2 and resistance level 3 for between 8 and 10 minutes, between 1 and 3 minutes on medium resistance and between 1 and 2 minutes on easy resistance. Shoot for between 25 and 30 minutes' total.

Week 2, Day 6 Abs and Legs

- *Barbell Squats:* Do 2 sets of between 10 and 12 repetitions if you can, do at least 1 set if possible.

- *Lunges with Dumbbells:* Do 2 sets of between 10 and 12 repetitions if you can, do at least 1 set if possible.

- *Sitting Leg Curls:* Do 2 sets of between 10 and 12 repetitions if you can, do at least 1 set if possible.

- *Barbell Deadlifts:* Do 2 sets of between 10 and 12 repetitions if you can, do at least 1 set if possible.

- *Sitting Calf Raises:* Do 2 sets of between 10 and 12 repetitions if you can, do at least 1 set if possible.

- *Calf Raises While Standing:* Do 2 sets of between 10 and 12 repetitions if you can, do at least 1 set if possible.

- *Crunches:* Do 2 sets of between 10 and 12 repetitions if you can, do at least 1 set if possible.

- *Leg Raises While Hanging:* Do 2 sets of between 10 and 12 repetitions if you can, do at least 1 set if possible.

Week 2, Day 7

- *Biceps and Back:* Do 2 sets of between 10 and 12 repetitions if you can, do at least 1 set if possible.

- *Pullups:* Do 2 sets of between 10 and 12 repetitions if you can, do at least 1 set if possible.

- *Back Extensions:* Do 2 sets of between 10 and 12 repetitions if you can, do at least 1 set if possible.

- *Concentrated Curls:* Do 2 sets of between 10 and 12 repetitions if you can, do at least 1 set if possible.

- *Barbell Curls:* Do 2 sets of between 10 and 12 repetitions if you can, do at least 1 set if possible.

- *Elliptical:* 1 or 2 minutes on an easy resistance, between 1 and 3 minutes on a moderate resistance, between 1 and 3 minutes on a difficult resistance, alternate between resistance level 2 and resistance level 3 for between 8 and 10 minutes, between 1 and 3 minutes on medium resistance and between 1 and 2 minutes on easy resistance. Shoot for between 25 and 30 minutes' total.

Keep it up

There you have it, the basic outline of the type of exercise plan you should get into the habit of following regularly. For the next two weeks, try and focus on improving the number of repetitions you complete each set and decreasing the extra time you spend resting.

The third set of two weeks should then be focused on maximizing your repetitions even more, with the goal of looking to increase the number of sets you are doing by 1, starting at the 8-week mark.

Remember, if you are anxious to build muscle as quickly as possible, the best way to do so is to aim for at least 10 repetitions with each set. This is the magic number when it comes to activating as much of your muscle tissue as possible. From that point on, each repetition you do is actively training your muscles as effectively as possible. Keep pushing yourself to do 1 more repetitions and the number of repetitions you can do will slowly but surely skyrocket.

While the first few weeks of regular exercise will likely lead to plenty of real results right off the bat, especially when coupled with the diet discussed in the following chapters, it is important to understand that you will not reach your goals overnight. Depending on how much work you have to do, it could be months, or maybe even years before you get the body of your dreams. While this may seem like an unfair slog, it is important to remember how long it took you to reach the point you were at before you started following a lean lifestyle and cut yourself some slack.

It is important to have a realistic level of expectation when it comes to the results you will see on the lean diet and not discount the methodical, if relatively unimpressive weekly returns that eating lean will bring you. However, week after week and month after month, if you stick with it, not only will you feel healthier and more full of energy than you ever thought possible, but you will eventually look in the mirror and hardly recognize the person looking back. Getting healthy is a marathon, not a sprint, slow and steady wins the race every time.

Chapter 3: Tips for Success and Mistakes to Avoid

Substitutions

When you first begin transitioning to a lean lifestyle, you may find that you routinely get cravings for specific types of foods that are now off of the table. One of the biggest reasons that many people fail to start a new diet once they have committed to it is they don't account for just how addictive many types of processed foods really are. Don't fall victim to the lure of unhealthy options, have a plan in place by keeping the following list in mind. The next time you get a craving, consider countering it in the following ways.

- Replace chocolate ice cream with chocolate flavored fat free Greek yogurt.

- Replace an ice cream sundae with frozen yogurt topped with fruit.

- Replace cheese doodles with non-processed cubes of actual cheese for a snack full of healthy fats.

- Replace chips and dip with vegetables and hummus.

- Replace a candy bar with a healthy protein bar.

- Replace potato chips with a small amount of air popped popcorn.

- Replace a cheese burger with a soy or black bean patty.

- Replace other salty favorites with healthy nut options instead.

In general, it is important to stay away from anything that is high in trans fats, sodium, sugar and hydrogenated oil. It is also important to try and limit your alcohol and soda and instead focus on drinking at least 12 cups of water per day. Both coffee and tea are acceptable as long as they are consumed black and not to excess.

Transitioning to a lean lifestyle

Unlike transitioning to many other diets, transitioning to a lean lifestyle can be relatively painless, depending on how committed you already are to eating primarily natural foods. If, however, you are heavily committed to processed foods, then you are in for an unfortunate couple of weeks. The high levels of fat and sugar that are found in most processed foods these days make many of them literally addictive.

This means that when you commit to cleaning out your refrigerator and going cold turkey with healthy alternatives you will feel the physical symptoms of withdrawal, the same as those detoxing from harmful drugs or alcohol. As such, you can either prepare for an unpleasant week or so whereby your body can experience flu like symptoms, or you can go cool turkey and try and wean yourself off of the unhealthier parts of your diet slowly to make the transition less painful.

If you make the decision to wean yourself off slowly, it is important to not try and follow the lean diet partially, and instead to work until you have gotten your sugar and fat consumption to a healthier point before committing to the new diet completely. Starting the lean diet partially is not recommended because of the dedication required when it comes to certain protein and healthy fat levels, something that cannot be guaranteed when processed foods are still in the mix. Don't give yourself an out when it comes to bailing on your new lifestyle prematurely, give it your all when you are in a position to do so.

Once you are ready to get started, it is important to do yourself a favor for later and take a number of "before" photographs and measurements to aid yourself in committing long term by proving yourself the opportunity to look back on how far you have come. This means you will want to weigh yourself on a scale as well as determine your current level of muscle mass and body fat. Don't forget to measure your shoulders, chest, waist, calves, thighs and arms for the best results.

While it may be difficult to look at yourself in such an analytical light, now, you will be happy in a few weeks' time when you have a baseline to compare your progress to. Write down your current measurements and put them someplace you will see them every morning, write down the new ones each time you take them and keep them in the same place. This visual representation of the timeline will make transitioning to the new lifestyle successfully much more manageable.

Sticking with a lean lifestyle

Once you have followed the outline provided in this book, you will need to make an effort set new goals for yourself if you hope to continue with the lean lifestyle in the long term. When choosing goals, it is important to choose those that are realistic to keep yourself from getting discouraged. This means losing between 1 and

1.5 lbs. per week in the long term while continuing to build muscle. Anything more than that is not just unrealistic, it is downright dangerous.

Instead of focusing on specific numbers on the scale, focus on increasing your number of repetitions or sets while exercising or how a specific item of clothing fits at different points in your journey. It is important to always have external factors working to push you in the right direction to keep your mind focused on the type of thought that will ensure you keep exercising regularly long enough for it to become a lifelong habit.

Likewise, it is important to be realistic about the fact that, now and then, you won't have the impregnable willpower required to stop yourself from eating something so delicious and so bad for you. If the healthy alternatives discussed above aren't enough to take your mind off of that one special something, it is instead a good idea to try and mitigate the damage as much as possible. Have 1, cupcake, not 20.

As long as you don't go crazy, there's no reason to feel guilty about the splurge afterwards, instead, take the time to think about how much healthier you are compared to when you started. The most important thing in these splurge scenarios is to not let the fact that you have gotten a little off book be the reason that you fall back into bad behavior. There is nothing wrong will a little splurge now and then, as long as you have the willpower to keep it an occasional thing.

Consider Carb Cycling

If you are looking to take the weight loss potential of your new lean lifestyle to the next level, you can consider adding carb cycling into the mix as well. Carb cycling is a separate type of dieting whereby you alternate the amount of carbohydrates you eat on certain days. Like the lean lifestyle, carb cycling focuses on eating clean foods and eating three large meals per day as well as two protein-rich snacks. It also promotes natural weight loss and lean muscle growth while improving your metabolism, all things that a lean lifestyle promotes as well.

Carb cycling works by ensuring you stock up on carbohydrates on your higher carbohydrate days to ensure you have the fuel you need to get you through the low carbohydrate days. Over time, this creates a scenario whereby your body starts burning a higher amount of calories on the higher carbohydrate days and then slowly begins to burn that higher amount of calories on the lower carbohydrate days which eventually become more and more frequent.

To get started carb cycling, you can start out alternating the days you can eat a higher amount of carbohydrates and the days you eat a smaller amount of carbohydrates and on each of the high amount of carbohydrates days you can eat a splurge item as long as you don't eat it in the evening. Starting on Monday, alternate between low and high carbohydrate days and allow both Saturday and Sunday to be higher carbohydrate days. On the low carbohydrate days, stick with 15 net grams of carbohydrates per day. Net carbohydrates are your total number of carbohydrates minus the amount of fiber you consume in the same day.

From there you can move on to a more standard, low/high split with Sunday being the only day that allows a splurge item. If you are looking to lose weight even faster you can double, or even triple up the ratio of lower carb to higher carb days as well.

When it comes to syncing carb cycling up with the rest of your schedule, it is important to ensure that the days you are eating the most carbohydrates are also the days that you are exercising the most stringently. Your body naturally needs more carbohydrates when exercising heavily anyway, might as well start putting all those extra carbs to good use right away. Don't forget to decrease the amount of healthy fat you eat on high carbohydrate days to balance things out.

Remember, just because you have the carbohydrate green light, doesn't mean you can eat unhealthy carbohydrates, instead you should stick to those that are complex which generate energy over a longer period of time. Reach for sweet potatoes, brown rice and dark, leafy vegetables and whatever you do, avoid high fructose corn syrup at all costs. Fructose is much more difficult for your muscles to utilize for energy which means it is much more likely that it will ultimately get stored as fat before a use for it is found.

Chapter 4: Week 1

Day 1

Breakfast

    Eggs (3 scrambled)

    Grapefruit (1 large)

Snack

    Almonds (25)

Lunch

    Turkey Wrap: This recipe requires 5 minutes to prepare and serves 1

        What's in It

- Flour tortilla (1)
- Hummus (2 T)
- Turkey (2 slices)
- Cucumber (.25 sliced)
- Tomato (.25 sliced)
- Red Onion (.25 sliced)

        How's it made

- Combine ingredients as desired serve and enjoy

Snack

Box of raisins (2 small)

Dinner

Side Salad with vinegar/olive oil (2 T)

Pasta and Spicy Chicken: This recipe requires 8 minutes to prepare, 10 minutes to cook and serves 4.

What's in It

- Angel hair pasta (9 oz.)
- Onion (1 cup sliced)
- Dried basil (1 T)
- Parmesan cheese (1 T grated)
- Spinach (10 oz. chopped)
- Chicken breast (6 oz.)
- Black pepper (to taste)
- Salt (to taste)
- Flour (1 tsp.)
- Sour cream (.25 cups)
- Half and half (1 cup)
- Red pepper (.5 tsp. crushed)
- Garlic (1.5 tsp. minced)

How's It Made

- Cook pasta as directed, minus any extra salt or fats. Drain the pasta but make sure to save .25 cups of liquid.
- Coat a skillet and place it on the stove over a burner turned to a high/medium heat.
- Add in the onion and let it cook for 2 minutes before adding in the garlic, red

pepper and basil and let everything cook an additional minute.

- In a bowl, combine the flour, sour cream and half and half and mix well.
- Add the results and the reserved liquid to the skillet and let it boil before adding in the remaining ingredients except the pasta and letting everything boil.
- Add in the pasta and let it heat to the desired temperature.

Day 2

Breakfast

Toast (1 piece)

Peanut Butter (2 T)

Snack

Box of raisins (2 small)

Lunch

Chicken Sausage with Peppers: This recipe requires 10 minutes of preparation, 10 minutes to cook and serves 4

What's in It

- Black Pepper (to taste)
- Salt (to taste)
- Basil (.25 cups chopped)
- Marinara sauce (1 cup)
- Worcestershire sauce (1 tsp.)
- Bell peppers (2 sliced)
- Red onion (1 sliced)

- Chicken sausage (1 lb.)
- Olive oil (1 T)

How's it Made

- Add the oil to a skillet before placing the skillet on the stove over a burner set to a high/medium heat.
- Add in the peppers and onions, season as desired and let them cook for 5 minutes.
- Add in the tomato sauce and the Worcestershire Sauce and letting everything cook for an additional 5 minutes. The sausage should be well cooked and the vegetables should be tender
- Top with basil prior to serving.

Snack

Fat free Greek yogurt (1 serving)

Dinner

Broccoli (2 cups)

Miso Salmon: This recipe requires 15 minutes of preparation, 10 minutes to cook and serves 4

What's in It

- Scallions (2 T)
- Salmon fillet (1.25 lbs. portioned)
- Hot pepper sauce (to taste)
- Ginger (1 T minced)
- Tamari (1 T)
- Mirin (2 T)
- Miso paste (2 T)

- Sesame seeds (1 T)

How's It Made

- Ensure your broiler is heated and place the oven rack in the top part of the oven.
- Prepare a baking pan by lining it with tinfoil and covering the foil with cooking spray.
- Place the sesame seeds into a skillet and place the skillet on a burner turned to a low heat and let them cook for 3 minutes, stirring all the while.
- In a small bowl, combine the hot pepper sauce, ginger, tamari, soy sauce, mirin and miso and mix well.
- Add the fish to the baking pan with the skin facing the foil. Coat well using the sauce before broiling the fish for about 7 minutes or until it is opaque in the middle.
- Top with scallions and sesame seeds before serving.

Day 3

Breakfast

Eggs (2)

Ham (1 slice)

Snack

Almonds (25)

Lunch

White Beans with Pesto and Asparagus: This recipe requires 15 minutes of preparation, 10 minutes to cook and serves 4.

What's in It-Pesto

- Black Pepper (to taste)
- Salt (to taste)
- Extra virgin olive oil (.25 cups)
- Lime juice (1 T)
- Parmesan cheese (.25 cups grated)
- Garlic (1 clove)
- Cilantro leaves (1 cup chopped)

What's in it-meal

- Coconut oil (1 T)
- Cherry tomatoes (1 cup sliced)
- Asparagus (1 lb. chopped)
- White beans (2 cups)

How's it Made

- To form the pesto, simply add the cilantro leaves, garlic, parmesan cheese, lime juice, extra virgin olive oil, and salt and pepper to a food processor and process well.
- Add the remaining coconut oil to a skillet before placing the skillet on the stove over a burner set to a high/medium heat.
- Add in the asparagus and let it cook until it has softened before mixing in the beans and letting everything cook for 5 minutes.
- Mix in the cherry tomatoes and let everything cook for 2 more minutes before adding in the pesto and cooking for 3 additional minutes.

Snack

>String cheese (1)

Dinner

>Side Salad with vinegar and olive oil (4 T)

>Sweet Potato Fries (1 serving)

>Veggie Burger with Whole Wheat Bun: This recipe requires 45 minutes to prepare, 30 minutes to cook and serves 8.

>>*What's in It*

>>- Low sodium soy sauce (1 T)
>>- Rolled oats (.3 cups quick cooking)
>>- Pecans (.5 cups toasted, chopped)
>>- Low fat cheddar cheese (.6 cups shredded)
>>- Egg (1)
>>- Oregano (.25 tsp. dried)
>>- Marjoram (.75 tsp. dried)
>>- Garlic (1 tsp. minced)
>>- White button mushrooms (2 cups chopped)
>>- Onion (1 cup diced)
>>- Canola oil (1 T)
>>- Red quinoa (.5 cups)
>>- Water (1 cup)

>>*How's It Made*

>>- In a saucepan, mix the quinoa and the water before placing the saucepan on the stove and letting it boil. Once it does so, cover it and let it simmer for 15 minutes. Once it is finished

- cooking, let it sit for 10 minutes, fluff as needed.
- Ensure your oven is heated to 350 degrees Fahrenheit.
- Cover a baking sheet in parchment paper.
- Add oil to a larger saucepan before placing it on top of a burner turned to a medium heat.
- Cook the onion in the saucepan for 5 minutes before adding in the oregano, marjoram, garlic and mushrooms and let everything cook an additional 5 minutes.
- While the second saucepan is cooling, beat the egg in a mixing bowl and then add in the soy sauce, oats, pecans, cheese, mushroom mix and quinoa and mix well.
- Portion out the results into .5 cup servings and place these servings onto the baking sheet before forming them into patties, leaving room for each to expand.
- Place the patties into the microwave and let them bake for 30 minutes

Day 4

Breakfast

Toast (1 slice)

Peanut Butter (2 T)

Fat Free Greek Yogurt (1 serving)

Snack

Snap Peas (15)

Hummus (2 T)

Lunch

Chicken Salad Lettuce Wraps: This recipe requires 10 minutes of preparation, 20 minutes to chill and serves 4

What's in It

- Black Pepper (to taste)
- Salt (to taste)
- Lettuce (4 large leaves)
- Low Fat balsamic vinaigrette (1 cup)
- Fat free Greek Yogurt (2 T plain)
- Cranberries (.25 cups dried)
- Grapes (.5 cups chopped)
- Walnuts (.5 cups toasted)
- Chicken (3 cups cooked, chopped)

How's it Made

- In a mixing bowl, combine the cranberries, grapes, walnuts and chicken and mix well before adding in the Greek yogurt and mixing thoroughly.
- Mix in the vinaigrette and season as desired before refrigerating for at least 20 minutes prior to serving.

Snack

1 Banana

Dinner

Broccoli (2 cups)

Brown rice (1 cup)

Snapper and Pesto: This recipe requires 10 minutes to prepare, 10 minutes to cook and serves 4.

What's in It

- Black pepper (to taste)
- Snapper (24 oz. fillets)
- Salt (.5 tsp.)
- Sugar (1 T)
- Garlic (3 cloves chopped)
- Lime juice (3 T)
- Olive oil (.25 cups)
- Mint leaves (.25 cups packed)
- Parsley (1.5 cups)
- Basil (1.5 cups)

How's It Made

- Add the salt, sugar, garlic, lime juice, oil, mint leaves, parsley and basil to a food processor and process well.
- Add the results to both sides of each fillet and use roughly .5 tsp. per side.
- Season as desired before placing the fish into a grill basket that has been prepared and letting the fish grill for 3.5 minutes on each side.

Day 5

Breakfast

Fat free Greek Yogurt (1 serving)

Grapefruit (1 large)

Snack

Protein Bar (1)

Lunch

1 apple

Lean Soufflé: This recipe requires 10 minutes of preparation, 2.5 minutes to cook and serves 4

What's in It

- Black Pepper (to taste)
- Salt (to taste)
- Rice Chex (1 handful crushed)
- Baby spinach (1 handful)
- Eggs (2)
- Extra virgin olive oil (1 T)

How's it Made

- Add the oil to a ramekin and coat well.
- Whisk the eggs together in a small bowl
- Add the crushed Chex to the ramekin and form a layer, follow it up with a layer of spinach and then top with the eggs.
- Stir briefly before adding the ramekin to the microwave and letting it cook for 1 minute before stirring again and letting it cook for another 1 minute and 30 seconds.
- Let cool for 5 minutes prior to eating.

Snack

Baby carrots (30)

Hummus (4 T)

Dinner

Snow peas (2 cups)

Brown rice (1 cup)

Spinach with Chicken Parmesan: This recipe requires 20 minutes of preparation, 20 minutes to cook and serves 6.

What's in It

- Whole-grain pasta (6 cups cooked, tossed with oil 2 tsp.)
- Mozzarella cheese (.75 cups shredded)
- Lemon juice (1 tsp.)
- Baby spinach (4 cups)
- Olive oil (2 T+2 tsp.)
- Chicken breast (1.5 lbs. portioned)
- Basil (.25 tsp. dried)
- Black pepper (.25 tsp. ground)
- Salt (.5 tsp. divided)
- Whole wheat flour (2 T)
- Parmesan cheese (3 T grated)
- Honey (.5 tsp.)
- Oregano (.25 tsp.)
- Basil (.25 tsp. dried)
- Whole tomatoes (28 oz.)
- Garlic (2 cloves sliced)
- Extra-virgin olive oil (2 tsp.)

How's It Made

- Ensure your oven is heated to 375 degrees Fahrenheit.
- Coat a baking pan in cooking spray.
- Place a saucepan on the stove over a burner turned to a medium heat before adding in the garlic and oil and letting the garlic cook for half a minute.
- Squeeze each tomato by hand into the pan before mixing in the honey, pepper, salt, oregano and basil. Simmer everything for approximately 20 minutes.
- Mix the basil, pepper, salt, flour and parmesan cheese together before using the results to cover the chicken.
- Add another skillet to the stove over a burner turned to a medium heat before adding in 2 T oil. After the oil begins to simmer, place the chicken in the skillet and cook one side for 6 minutes.
- Add the chicken to the baking pan
- Add the remaining oil to the skillet before adding in the spinach. Let it cook for 2 minutes before swirling in the lemon juice.
- Add the spinach to the top of the chicken and top with sauce and cheese.
- Place the baking pan in the oven and let it cook for 15 minutes.

Day 6

Breakfast

> Eggs (2)
>
> Vegetable (1)
>
> Banana (1)

Snack

> String cheese (1)

Lunch

> Sesame Tofu, Scallion and Ginger: This recipe requires 10 minutes of preparation, 5 minutes to cook and serves 2.

> *What's in It*
>
> - Extra-virgin olive oil (2 tsp.)
> - Salt (to taste)
> - Black pepper (to taste)
> - Smoked paprika (1 tsp.)
> - Sesame seeds (2 T)
> - Scallions (.25 cups diced)
> - Ginger (2 tsp.)
> - Tofu (1 cup diced)

> *How's It Made*
>
> - Add the oil to a skillet and place the skillet on the stove over a burner set to a high/medium heat.
> - Add in the scallions as well as the ginger and let them cook for 60 seconds before mixing in the tofu and scrambling it.

- Let the tofu cook completely before removing it from the burner and mixing in the smoked paprika, sesame seed and any salt or pepper as desired.

Snack

Cherry Tomatoes (10)

Hummus (2 T)

Dinner

Broccoli (2 cups)

Brown rice (1 cup)

Lemon Chicken with Dill: This recipe requires 30 minutes of active cooking time and serves 4

What's in It

- Lemon juice (1 T)
- Dill (2 T chopped, divided)
- Flour (2 tsp.)
- Low sodium chicken broth (1 cup)
- Garlic (3 cloves minced)
- Onion (.25 cups chopped)
- Extra-virgin olive oil (3 tsp. divided)
- Black pepper (to taste)
- Salt (to taste)

- Chicken breast (1.25 lbs. portioned)

How's It Made

- Add seasoning to the chicken as desired.
- Add 1.5 tsp. of oil to a skillet before placing it on the stove over a burner turned to a high/medium heat. Place the chicken in the skillet and cook each side for 3 minutes. Remove the chicken from the skillet and cover it with foil.
- Turn the burner heat to medium before adding in the rest of the oil as well as garlic and onion before stirring and cooking for 1 minute.
- Combine the lemon juice, dill, flour and broth together before adding the results to the pan and letting everything cook for 3 minutes.
- Add the chicken back to the pan before turning the burner to low and letting everything simmer for 4 minutes.
- Season the sauce as desired and top the chicken with it prior to serving.

Day 7

Breakfast

Eggs (2)

Vegetable (1)

Banana (1)

Snack

Baby carrots (15)

Hummus (2 T)

Lunch

Mango Salsa and Pork Tenderloin: Sesame Tofu, Scallion and Ginger: This recipe requires 15 minutes of preparation, 25 minutes to cook and serves 4.

What's in It-Pork

- Extra-virgin olive oil (2 T divided)
- Salt (to taste)
- Black pepper (to taste)
- Pork tenderloin (1.25 lbs.)
- Jerk seasoning (2 T)

What's in It-Salsa

- Lime (1 quartered)
- Salt (to taste)
- Jalapeno (2 tsp. diced)
- Lime juice (1 T)
- Cilantro (.25 cups)
- Red onion (.25 cups)
- Mango (.5 cups)
- Pineapple (1 cup)

How's It Made

- Mix the salt, jerk seasoning and 1 T extra virgin olive oil in a small bowl before coating the pork in the results.
- Place the pork in a sealable plastic bag with the leftover marinade and let it sit in the refrigerator for 30 minutes.

- Combine the pineapple, mango, red onion, cilantro, lime juice, jalapeno and salt together in a food processor and process as desired.
- After the pork has finished marinating, leave it at room temperature to warm for about 15 minutes.
- Add the oil to a skillet and place the skillet on the stove over a burner set to a high/medium heat.
- Once it has warmed completely, add in the pork and let it cook until it is browned on both sides, roughly 2 minutes per side.
- Cover the pan with tinfoil and reduce the heat and continue to let it cook until the internal temperature of the pork reaches 145 degrees Fahrenheit.
- Let the pork cool for 3 minutes prior to serving, top with salsa as desired and garnish with the lime wedge.

Snack

Fat free Greek yogurt (1 serving)

Dinner

Broccoli (2 cups)

Chicken Marengo and Penne: This recipe requires 20 minutes of preparation, 15 minutes to cook and makes 4 servings.

What's in It

- Butter (.5 T)
- Tomatoes (14 oz. chopped)
- Beef broth (.5 cups)

- White wine (.5 cups)
- Tomato paste (2 T)
- Yellow bell pepper (1 seeded, julienned)
- Mushrooms (.5 lbs. sliced)
- Sweet onion (1 sliced)
- Vegetable oil (3 T)
- Flour (.5 cups)
- Black pepper (to taste)
- Salt (to taste)
- Chicken cutlets (3 thinly sliced)

How's It Made

- Season the chicken as desired before coating it in flour.
- Add the oil to a sauté pan before placing the pan over a burner turned to a high/medium heat before adding in the chicken and let it brown for 3 minutes per side.
- Once the chicken has finished browning completely, remove it from the pan before adding in additional oil and mixing in the peppers, mushrooms and onion and letting the cook for 5 minutes, seasoning as needed.
- Mix in the tomato paste, and let it cook for 2 minutes before increasing the heat, mixing in the wine and letting it reduce for 2 minutes.
- Mix in the tomatoes as well as the beef broth and let it start to bubble before mixing in the chicken and letting everything simmer for 3 minutes.
- Before serving, stir in the butter.

Chapter 5: Week 2

Day 1

Breakfast

> Scrambled eggs (3)
>
> Grapefruit (1 large)

Snack

> Almonds (25)

Lunch

> Chicken Curry Pita: This recipe requires 15 minutes of active cooking time and serves 4.
>
> *What's in It*
>
> - Sprouts (2 cups)
> - Pita (4 5-inch, cut in half)
> - Almonds (.25 cups sliced, toasted)
> - Cranberries (.5 cups dried)
> - Celery (1 stalk diced fine)
> - Pear (1 diced)
> - Chicken breast (2 cups cubed)
> - Curry powder (1 T)
> - Low-fat mayonnaise (.25 cups)
> - Fat free plain Greek yogurt (6 T)
>
> *How's It Made*

- In a large bowl, mix the curry powder, mayonnaise and yogurt together before adding in the almonds, cranberries, celery, pear and chicken, mix well and season as desired.
- Add the results to the pita and top with sprouts.

Snack

String cheese (1 piece)

Fat free Greek Yogurt (1 serving)

Dinner

Snow peas (2 cups)

Asian Lettuce Wraps: This recipe requires 5 minutes of preparation, 10 minutes to cook and makes 4 servings.

What's in It

- Lime (1 wedged)
- Cilantro (1 bunch dried)
- Mint (1 bunch (dried)
- Cucumber (1 peeled, sliced thin)
- Lettuce (12 leaves)
- Sesame oil (1 tsp.)
- Soy sauce (3 T)
- Sugar (1 tsp.)
- Red pepper flakes (.5 tsp.)
- Garlic (2 cloves chopped)
- Ginger (2 T chopped)
- Scallions (3 sliced)
- Red pepper (1 seeded, sliced)

- Ground beef (1 lb.)
- Vegetable oil (1 T)

How's It Made

- Add the oil to a skillet before placing the skillet on the stove over a burner turned to a high/medium heat. Crumble the beef and add it to the skillet to cook for 5 minutes.
- Add in the sugar, red pepper flakes, garlic, ginger, scallion and red pepper. Turn the heat off and mix in the sesame oil and soy sauce.
- Combine ingredients as desired prior to serving.

Day 2

Breakfast

Eggs (2)

Vegetable (1)

String cheese (1)

Snack

Fat free Greek Yogurt (1 serving)

1 banana

Lunch

Salmon Sammie: This recipe requires 15 minutes of preparation and serves 4.

What's in It

- Extra-virgin olive oil (1 T)

- Salt (to taste)
- Black pepper (to taste)
- Romaine lettuce (2 large leaves, halved)
- Tomato (8 slices)
- Pumpernickel bread (8 slices toasted)
- Low fat cream cheese (4 T)
- Lemon juice (2 T)
- Red onion (.25 cups minced)
- Salmon (14 oz.)

How's It Made

- In a mixing bowl, combine the oil, lemon juice, onion and salmon, mix well and season as desired.
- Spread 1 T of the cream cheese on half of the bread slices and then cover this with .5 cups of salmon salad.
- Top with 2 slices of tomato and the remaining bread.

Snack

Cherry tomatoes (10)

Hummus (2 T)

Dinner

Brown Rice (1 cup)

Broccoli (2 cups)

Tofu and Broccoli Stir Fry: This recipe requires 30 minutes of active cooking time and makes 4 servings.

What's in It

- Water (3 T)
- Broccoli florets (6 cups)
- Ginger (1 T minced)
- Extra virgin olive oil (2 T divided)
- Salt (.25 tsp.)
- Tofu (14 oz. drained)
- Red pepper flakes (.25 tsp.)
- Sugar (2 T + 1 tsp.)
- Cornstarch (3 T divided)
- Low sodium soy sauce (3 T)
- Dry sherry (.25 cups)
- Vegetable broth (.5 cups)

How's It Made

- In a small bowl, mix the soy sauce, sherry, the broth, red pepper flakes, sugar and 1 T corn starch and combine well.
- Cube tofu and season as desired.
- In a large bowl, place the remainder of the cornstarch before adding in the tofu and coating well.
- Add 1 T oil to a pan and place the pan on the stove over a burner turned to a high/medium heat. Mix in the tofu and let it brown completely.
- Remove the tofu from the skillet before turning the heat to medium and adding in the rest of the oil as well as the ginger and garlic and let it cook for 30 seconds. Add in the water as well as the broccoli before covering the skillet and letting it cook for 3 minutes, stirring regularly.

- Add in the broth mixture and let it thicken for 1 minute.
- Combine all ingredients prior to serving.

Day 3

Breakfast

    Eggs (3 scrambled)

    Grapefruit (1 large)

Snack

    Fat free Greek yogurt (1 serving)

    Almonds (25)

Lunch

Charred Tomato, Broccoli and Chicken Salad: This recipe requires 40 minutes of preparation, 20 minutes to cook and serves 6.

What's in It

- Extra-virgin olive oil (2 tsp. + 3T)
- Salt (to taste)
- Black pepper (to taste)
- Lemon juice (.25 cups)
- Chili powder (.5 tsp.)
- Tomatoes (1.5 lbs. halved)
- Broccoli (4 cups florets)
- Chicken breast (1.5 lbs.)

How's It Made

- Add the chicken to a saucepan and fill the saucepan with water so the chicken is covered.
- Add the saucepan to the stove over a burner set to a high heat and let the water simmer. Once it does, cover the pan, reduce the heat and let it cook for 12 minutes.
- Once the chicken has cooled enough to handle, shred it.
- Add a large pot of water to the stove over a burner set to a high heat. After it boils, add in the broccoli and let it cook for 3 minutes.
- Drain the broccoli and refill the pot with cool water.
- Place the skillet on the stove over a burner set to a high heat and coat the halved side of the tomato in oil before placing them in the skillet.
- Let the tomatoes cook for 4 minutes before topping with more oil and charring the other sides as well.
- Remove the tomatoes from the skillet and chop them.
- Add the remaining oil to the skillet without cleaning the skill and mix in the chili powder, pepper and salt and letting them cook for about 30 seconds. Add in the lemon juice and take the pan off of the burner.
- Add the results to a large bowl and mix in the broccoli, chicken and the tomatoes and combine well.

Snack

String cheese (1)

Banana (1)

Dinner

Broccoli (2 cups)

Sour and Sweet Chicken and Brown Rice: This recipe requires about 30 minutes of active cooking time and makes 4 servings.

What's in It

- Water chestnuts (5 oz. drained, sliced)
- Vegetable medley (6 cups)
- Low sodium chicken broth (1 cup)
- Ginger (2 tsp. minced)
- Garlic (4 cloves minced)
- Chicken tenders (1 lb. halved)
- Extra virgin olive oil (2 T)
- Apricot preserves (2 T)
- Cornstarch (2 T)
- Low sodium soy sauce (2 T)
- Rice vinegar (.25 cups)
- Instant brown rice (2 cups prepared)

How's It Made

- In a small bowl, combine the apricot preserves, cornstarch, soy sauce and vinegar and whisk well.
- Add 1 T oil to a skillet before placing the skillet on the stove over a burner set to a high/medium heat. Place the chicken in the skillet and let it cook for 2 minutes. After two minutes, stir and then let it cook for an additional 2 minutes. Remove the chicken from the skillet.

- Add the rest of the oil to the pan before adding in the ginger and garlic and letting them cook for 20 seconds. Mix in the broth and stir while waiting for it to boil. Mix in the vegetables before letting it simmer. Cover the skillet and let everything cook for 4 minutes.
- Add in the chicken and the water chestnuts before adding in the sauce. Let it thicken for 1 minute and mix with rice prior to serving.

Day 4

Breakfast

Toast (1 slice)

Peanut Butter (2 T)

Snack

Raisins (2 small boxes)

Lunch

Sun Dried Tomato, Corn and Turkey Wrap: This recipe requires 20 minutes of preparation and serves 4.

What's in It

- Extra-virgin olive oil (2 T)
- Salt (to taste)
- Black pepper (to taste)
- Romaine Lettuce (2 cups)
- Whole wheat tortillas (4)
- Turkey (8 oz. sliced)
- Red wine vinegar (1 T)
- Sun-dried tomatoes (.25 cups chopped)

- Tomato (.5 cups chopped)
- Corn (1 cup kernels)

How's It Made

- In a mixing bowl, combine the red wine vinegar, the extra virgin olive oil, the sun dried tomatoes, the regular tomatoes and the corn and mix well.
- Add the turkey and lettuce to the tortillas before filling them with the mixture from the bowl.

Snack

Protein bar (1)

Dinner

Broccoli (2 cups)

Brown Rice (1 cup)

Chicken with Lime and Cilantro: This recipe requires 10 minutes of preparation, 40 minutes to cook and makes 8 servings.

What's in It

- Cilantro (.25 cups chopped)
- Lime juice (2 limes)
- Low sodium chicken broth (1 cup)
- Garlic (2 cloves minced)
- Unsalted butter (4 T divided)
- Black pepper (to taste)
- Salt (to taste)
- Paprika (1 tsp.)

- Basil (1 tsp. dried)
- Oregano (2 tsp. dried)
- Chicken thighs (8)
- Brown sugar (8 tsp. divided)

How's It Made

- Ensure you oven is heated to 400 degrees Fahrenheit.
- Coat the chicken with a mixture of sugar, pepper, salt, paprika, basil and oregano.
- Add 2 T butter to a skillet before placing the skillet on the stove over a burner turned to a high/medium heat. Place the chicken in the skillet with the skin touching the skillet and sear each side for approximately 2 minutes until browned.
- Drain the fat from the skillet and remove the chicken from the skillet.
- Add the rest of the butter to the skillet before adding in the garlic and letting it cook for 1 minute, stirring regularly. Add in the broth, cilantro and lime juice before letting it boil and then turning the heat down and letting it simmer for 5 minutes.
- Add the chicken back into the skillet before placing the skillet in the oven and letting it cook for about 25 minutes or until the center of the chicken reaches 165 degrees Fahrenheit.

Day 5

Breakfast

> Eggs (2)
>
> Vegetable (1)
>
> Grapefruit (1 large)

Snack

> Fat Free Greek Yogurt (1 serving)
>
> Banana (1)

Lunch

> Crab Roll: This recipe requires 20 minutes of preparation and serves 4.

> ### *What's in It*
>
> - Salt (to taste)
> - Black pepper (to taste)
> - Whole wheat pita (4)
> - Red lettuce (4 leaves)
> - Crabmeat (2 cups cooked)
> - Chives (.25 cups sliced, divided)
> - Celery (.25 cups chopped)
> - Shallot (.25 cups chopped)
> - Hot sauce (10 dashes)
> - Lemon juice (3 T)
> - Lemon zest (1 T grated)
> - Fat free mayonnaise (.25 cups)

> ### *How's It Made*

- In a mixing bowl, combine the salt, pepper, hot sauce, lemon juice, lemon zest and mayonnaise together and whisk well.
- Add in 3 T chives, celery and shallot and mix well before adding in the crab and mixing gently.
- Add the lettuce to the pita and fill each with the crab mixture, top with the remaining chives.

Snack

Baby carrots (15)

Hummus (2 T)

Dinner

Brown rice (1 cup)

Broccoli (2 cups)

Dill Sauce and Salmon: This recipe requires 15 minutes of preparation time and makes 4 servings.

What's in It

- Capers (1 T chopped)
- Dill (2 T chopped)
- Lemon juice (2 T)
- Sour cream (.5 cups)
- Green beans (1 lb. trimmed)
- Black pepper (to taste)
- Salt (to taste)
- Salmon fillet (24 oz. portioned)
- Extra Virgin Olive Oil (1 T)

How's It Made

- Add the oil to your skillet before placing the skillet on the stove over a medium heat.
- Season the salmon as desired before adding it to the skillet and letting it cook for 5 minutes on each side and ensuring the center is opaque.
- While the fish is cooking, place a steamer basket into a saucepan and let 1 inch of water in the pan begin to boil. Add the beans and cover the pot to let them cook for 4 minutes.
- Mix together the capers, dill, lemon juice, sour cream and pepper and salt as desired and top the salmon prior to serving.

Day 6

Breakfast

Ham (1 slice)

Eggs (2)

Grapefruit (1 medium)

Snack

Almonds (25)

String cheese (1)

Lunch

White Bean Salad with Chicken: This recipe requires 25 minutes of preparation and serves 4.

What's in It-Salad

- Salt (to taste)
- Black pepper (to taste)

- Radicchio leaves (2 cups torn)
- Romaine lettuce (2 cups torn)
- Basil (1 cup chopped coarse)
- Sun dried tomatoes (.3 cups chopped)
- Feta cheese (.25 cups diced)
- Celery (1.5 cups diced)
- Zucchini (2 cups diced)
- Chicken breast (2.5 cups diced)
- White beans (15 oz.)

What's in It-Vinaigrette

- Dijon mustard (1 T)
- White wine vinegar (.25 cups)
- Orange juice (6 T)
- Extra virgin olive oil (5 T)
- Salt (.25 tsp.)
- Garlic (1 clove peeled, smashed)

How's It Made

- To create the vinaigrette, start by mashing the garlic along with .25 tsp. salt in a small bowl to create a paste.
- Add in 5 T oil and mix well before mixing in the orange juice, mustard, vinegar and combine thoroughly. Add up to 4 more Tablespoons of juice to cut the flavor as needed.
- In a large bowl, combine the sun dried tomatoes, cheese, celery, zucchini, chicken and white beans and mix well. Add in .75 cups vinaigrette and the basil, season as needed and mix well.

- Add all of the ingredients to a salad bowl and mix well prior to serving.

Snack

Cherry Tomatoes (10)

Hummus (2 T)

Dinner

Broccoli (2 cups)

Poblanos Stuffed with Barley: This recipe requires 10 minutes of preparation, 55 minutes to cook and makes 6 servings.

What's in It

- Queso fresco (.5 cups crumbled)
- Low fat Monterey Jack cheese (3 slices halved)
- Low fat white cheddar (2 oz. grated)
- Poblano peppers (6 large)
- Slat (.25 tsp.)
- Whole peeled tomatoes (28 oz. crushed)
- Garlic (3 cloves minced)
- Chili powder (1 tsp. divided)
- Kale (1 bunch chopped)
- Barley (1.5 cups soaked, drained)
- Onion (1 diced)
- Extra virgin olive oil (3 T)

How's It Made

- Add 1 T oil to a saucepan and place it over a burner turned to a medium heat. Place the onion in the pan and let it cook for 5 minutes before adding in 3.75 cups water and the barley and letting it cook for 30 minutes before adding in the cheddar cheese, kale and half of the chili powder.

- While the barely is cooking, place the rest of the oil into a heavy pot before placing the pot on the stove over a burner turned to a medium heat. Add in the garlic and let it cook for 3 minutes before adding in the tomatoes, the rest of the chili powder and the salt before letting the pot boil. Let the pot simmer for 30 minutes, covered on a low heat.
- Ensure your broiler is heated and positioned in the middle of the oven.
- Cut the tops off of the peppers and remove the innards but save the tops. Add the barley mix to the peppers and place the tops back on before placing them in a baking dish and broiling them for 20 minutes, turning at the 10-minute mark.
- At this point, put the tomato sauce in the pan as well. Add .5 slices of the Monterey Jack cheese to the top of each pepper. Melt the cheese by broiling for 1 minute.
- Top with queso fresco prior to serving.

Day 7

Breakfast

Toast (1 slice)

Peanut butter (2 T)

Grapefruit (1 large)

Snack

>Raisins (2 small boxes)

>String cheese (1)

Lunch

>Tarragon chicken salad: This recipe requires 15 minutes of preparation, 30 minutes to cook and serves 8.

>### *What's in It*

>- Salt (to taste)
>- Black pepper (to taste)
>- Red grapes (1.5 cups halved)
>- Celery (1.5 cups sliced)
>- Tarragon (1 T)
>- Fat free mayonnaise (.5 cups)
>- Low fat sour cream (.6 cups)
>- Walnuts (.3 cups chopped)
>- Low sodium chicken broth (1 cup)
>- Chicken breast (2 lbs.)

>### *How's It Made*

>- Ensure your oven is heated to 450 degrees Fahrenheit.
>- Place the chicken into a glass baking dish so that it is spread in a single layer and then add in the broth.
>- Let the chicken bake for 30 minutes or until its internal temperature reads 170 degrees Fahrenheit.
>- Cube the chicken once it has cooled.

- Place the walnuts onto a baking sheet and toast them in the oven for approximately 6 minutes before letting them cool.
- In a mixing bowl, combine the pepper, salt, tarragon, mayonnaise and sour cream together before adding in the walnuts, chicken, grapes and celery and coating well.
- Chill for 1 hour prior to serving.

Snack

Baby carrots (15)

Hummus (2 T)

Dinner

Side salad with vinegar and olive oil (2 T)

Baja Fish Tacos: This recipe requires 5 minutes of preparation, 8 minutes to cook and makes 4 servings.

What's in It

- Limes (2 wedged)
- Salsa (to taste)
- Avocado (.5 diced, pitted)
- Corn tortillas (8)
- Cilantro (3 T)
- Salt (.5 tsp.)
- Lime juice (1 T)
- Green cabbage (2 cups sliced)
- Fajita seasoning (2 tsp.)
- Mahi Mahi (.75 lbs.)

How's It Made

- Prepare the grill and heat it to a medium heat.
- Season the fish as desired before adding it to the grill and letting each side cook for 3 minutes.
- Combine the cilantro, salt, lime juice and cabbage together in a bowl.
- Combine all ingredients prior to serving.

Chapter 6: Week 3

Day 1

Breakfast

> Eggs (2)
>
> Vegetable (1)
>
> Grapefruit (1 large)

Snack

> Cherry Tomatoes (10)
>
> Hummus (2 T)

Lunch

> Tofu Peanut Wrap: This recipe requires 10 minutes of preparation and serves 1.
>
> > *What's in It*
> >
> > - Snow peas (8 sliced)
> > - Red bell pepper (.25 cups sliced)
> > - Tofu (2 oz. baked, sliced)
> > - Wheat tortilla (1)
> > - Peanut Sauce (1 T)
> >
> > *How's It Made*
> >
> > - . Add all of the ingredients to the tortilla, wrap and serve.

Snack

Fat free Greek yogurt (1 serving)

Dinner

Broccoli (2 cups)

Fettuccine with Peas and Shrimp: This recipe requires 10 minutes of preparation, 1 minutes to cook and makes 3 servings.

What's in It

- Parmesan cheese (to taste)
- Peas (3 T)
- Rosemary (.5 tsp. crushed)
- Garlic (1 tsp. minced)
- Tomatoes (.25 cups chopped)
- Shrimp (.3 cups)
- Extra Virgin olive oil (1 T)
- Whole wheat pasta (1 package prepared)

How's It Made

- Add the oil to a skillet before adding in the rosemary, garlic and tomatoes and letting them cook for 5 minutes, stirring twice per minute.
- Add in the peas and then cook and stir for 2 minutes.
- Combine all of the ingredients and top with the cheese prior to serving.

Day 2

Breakfast

Eggs (3 scrambled)

Grapefruit (1 large)

Snack

String cheese (1)

Lunch

Turkey Lettuce Wrap: This recipe requires 30 minutes of preparation and serves 6.

What's in It

- Sesame oil (2 tsp.)
- Salt (to taste)
- Black pepper (to taste)
- Carrot (1 shredded)
- Cilantro (.5 cups chopped)
- Basil (.5 cups chopped)
- Mint (.5 cups chopped)
- Boston lettuce (2 heads separated leaves)
- Five spice powder (1 tsp.)
- Hoisin sauce (2 T)
- Low sodium chicken broth (.5 cups reduced)
- Water chestnuts (8 oz. chopped)
- Red bell pepper (1 diced fine)
- Ginger (1 T minced)
- Ground turkey (1 lb.)
- Instant brown rice (.5 cups)
- Water (.5 cup)

How's It Made

- Fill a small saucepan with water and place it on the stove over a burner set to a high heat and let the water boil. Add in the rice and let it cook for 5 minutes and remove the saucepan from the burner.
- Add the oil to a skillet and place it on the stove over a burner set to a medium heat. Add in the ginger and crumble in the turkey before letting it cook for 6 minutes.
- Add in the rice, salt, pepper, five spice powder, hoisin sauce, broth, water chestnuts, mint, basil, cilantro, bell pepper and let everything cook for 1 minute.
- Add the turkey mix, carrots and herbs to each piece of lettuce and roll it like a burrito.

Snack

Almonds (25)

Dinner

Brown rice (1 cup)

Veggie Stir Fry: This recipe requires 15 minutes of preparation, 5 minutes to cook and makes 6 servings.

What's in It

- Sesame oil (2 T)
- Snow peas (.5 cups)
- Salt (.25 tsp.)
- Black pepper (.25 tsp.)
- Mung bean sprouts (1 cup)
- Bok choy (2 cups sliced)
- Teriyaki sauce (.5 cups)
- Garlic (1 clove minced)

- Eggplant (1 chopped)
- Broccoli (1 cup florets)
- Yellow squash (1 cup sliced)
- Red onion (.5 cups sliced thin)
- Yellow bell pepper (seeded, cored, julienned)
- Extra virgin olive oil (2 T)

How's It Made

- Add the oil to a skillet before adding the skillet to the stove over a burner turned to a high heat. Once the skillet is almost smoking, mix in the onion and peppers before adding in the garlic eggplant, broccoli, squash and the sauce.
- Stir for 2 minutes before adding in the seasoning, sprouts and bok choy and stirring for an additional 2 minutes.
- Remove the skillet from the heat and add in the sesame oil and snow peas prior to serving.

Day 3

Breakfast

Oatmeal (1 serving)

Grapefruit (1 large)

Snack

String cheese (1)

Lunch

Cobb Salad: This recipe requires 15 minutes of preparation, 25 minutes to cook and serves 4.

What's in It

- Extra-virgin olive oil (3 T)
- Salt (to taste)
- Black pepper (to taste)
- Blue cheese (.5 cups crumbles)
- Avocado (1 diced)
- Cucumber (1 sliced, seeded)
- Tomatoes (2 diced)
- Eggs (2)
- Cooked chicken breast (8 oz.)
- Salad greens (10 cups)
- Dijon mustard (1 T)
- Shallot (2 T minced)
- White wine vinegar (3 T)

How's It Made

- Start by poaching the chicken breast. Add it to a skillet before covering it in salted water. Add the skillet to the stove over a burner set to a high/medium heat and let it boil.
- Once it does, turn the burner to low and let it simmer for 10 minutes or until the chicken reaches 165 degrees Fahrenheit internally.
- Let the chicken cool and then shred it.
- Place the eggs in a saucepan and cover them with 1 inch of water. Add the pan to the stove over a burner set to a high/medium heat. Once the pan simmers, reduce the heat and let it slightly simmer 10 minutes.
- Drain the eggs and cover them with cool water. Once they have cooled, peel and chop them.

- In a small bowl, combine the salt, pepper, mustard, shallot and vinegar and mix well.
- In a large bowl, combine the salad greens with 50 percent of the dressing and coat well.
- Plate everything and top with the remaining dressing prior to serving.

Snack

Fat free Greek Yogurt (1 serving)

Dinner

Side salad with vinegar and olive oil (2 T)

Broccoli (2 cups)

Balsamic chicken: This recipe requires 10 minutes of preparation, 25 minutes to cook and makes 6 servings.

What's in It

- Thyme (.5 tsp. dried)
- Rosemary (1 tsp. dried)
- Oregano (1 tsp. dried)
- Basil (1 tsp. dried)
- Balsamic vinegar (.5 cups)
- Tomatoes (14.5 oz. diced)
- Onion (1 sliced thin)
- Extra virgin olive oil (2 T)
- Black pepper (to taste)
- Garlic salt (1 tsp.)
- Chicken breast (3 halved)

How's It Made

- Season the chicken as desired.

- Add the oil to the skillet before placing the skillet on the stove over a burner set to a medium heat. Add in the chicken and let it cook for 3 minutes per side.
- Add in the onion and let everything cook an additional 3 minutes.
- Add in the vinegar and tomatoes on top of the chicken before adding in the thyme, rosemary, oregano and basil. Let everything simmer for 15 minutes, the chicken should reach a temperature of 165 degrees Fahrenheit.

Day 4

Breakfast

Ham (1 slice)

Eggs (2)

Grapefruit (1 medium)

Snack

Fat Free Greek Yogurt

1 banana

Lunch

Tuna Panini: This recipe requires 25 minutes of preparation and serves 4.

What's in It

- Extra-virgin olive oil (2 tsp.)
- Salt (to taste)
- Black pepper (to taste)

- Wholegrain bread (8 slices)
- Lemon juice (1 tsp.)
- Capers (1 tsp. chopped)
- Kalamata olives (1 T chopped, pitted)
- Red onion (2 T minced)
- Artichoke hearts (2 T chopped)
- Feta cheese (.25 cups crumbled)
- Plum tomato (1 chopped)
- Light tuna (12 oz. chunked)

How's It Made

- Flake the tuna in a bowl with the help of a fork. Mix in the pepper, salt, lemon juice, capers, olives, onion, artichokes, feta and tomato and combine well.
- Place .5 cups of the tuna mixture on half of the slices. And top the sandwiches.
- Add the oil to a skillet and place the skillet on the stove over a burner set to a high/medium heat. Add 2 panni to the skillet at a time, and cook the first side for 2 minutes, reduce the heat to low/medium and cook the other side for 2 minutes.
- Add additional oil for the second set of sandwiches as needed.

Snack

String cheese (1)

Dinner

Broccoli (2 cups)

Brown rice (1 cup)

Swai Fillet: This recipe requires 10 minutes of preparation, 15 minutes to cook and makes 4 servings.

What's in It

- Paprika (1 tsp.)
- Black pepper (1 tsp.)
- Salt (1 tsp.)
- Garlic (1 tsp. minced)
- Cilantro (1 T)
- Lemon juice (1 T)
- Dry white wine (.25 cups)
- Margarine (2 T)
- Swai fish fillet (16 oz. portioned)

How's It Made

- Ensure your oven is heated to 350 degrees Fahrenheit.
- Coat a baking sheet in cooking spray and add in the fillets.
- Add the margarine to a saucepan before adding the pan to the stove over a burner turned to a medium heat. Add in the pepper, salt, garlic, cilantro, lemon juice and white wine and let it simmer for 2 minutes.
- Add in the paprika and ensure the fish is well covered in the sauce before adding the pan to the oven and letting it cook for 10 minutes.

Day 5

Breakfast

> Toast (1 slice)
>
> Peanut butter (2 T)
>
> Grapefruit (1 medium)

Snack

> Banana (1)
>
> Box of raisins (1 small)

Lunch

> Red Lentil Curry Soup: This recipe requires 15 minutes of preparation, 45 minutes to cook and serves 6.
>
> > *What's in It*
> >
> > - Extra-virgin olive oil (1 T)
> > - Salt (to taste)
> > - Black pepper (to taste)
> > - Fat free plain Greek yogurt (.3 cups)
> > - Mango chutney (2 T)
> > - Lemon juice (2 T)
> > - Cilantro (3 T)
> > - Low sodium chicken broth (8 cups)
> > - Red lentils (1.5 cups)
> > - Bay leaves (2)
> > - Cumin (1 tsp. ground)
> > - Cinnamon (1 tsp.)
> > - Curry powder (1.5 T)
> > - Jalapeno (1 seeded, minced)
> > - Ginger (2 T minced)
> > - Garlic (3 cloves minced)

- Onion (1 chopped)

How's It Made

- Add the oil to a stockpot and place the pot on the stove over a burner set to a medium heat. Add in the onion and let it cook for 3 minutes before adding in the bay leaves, cumin, cinnamon, curry powder, jalapeno, ginger and garlic. Stir and let it cook for 5 minutes.
- Add in the chicken broth as well as the lentils and let the pot boil before turning the heat to low, covering the pot part way and letting it simmer for 45 minutes.
- Remove the bay leaves and add in the cilantro, chutney and lemon juice before seasoning as desired.
- Add the yogurt to each bowl prior to serving.

Snack

Baby carrots (15)

Hummus (2 T)

Dinner

Side salad with vinegar and olive oil (2 T)

Bean Quesadilla: This recipe requires 15 minutes of active preparation time and makes 4 servings.

What's in It

- Avocado (1 diced)
- Extra virgin olive oil (2 tsp.)
- Whole wheat tortillas (4)

- Salsa (.5 cups)
- Monterey Jack cheese (.5 cups shredded)
- Black beans (15 oz.)

How's It Made

- In a mixing bowl, combine .25 cups salsa with the Monterey Jack cheese and the black beans before mixing well.
- Add the results to the tortillas before folding them in half.
- Add 1 tsp. of extra virgin olive oil to a skillet and place the skillet on the stove over an oven turned to a medium heat. Cook each side of each quesadilla for 2 minutes. 1 tsp. of olive oil will cook 2 quesadillas.

Day 6

Breakfast

Eggs (3 scrambled)

Grapefruit (1 large)

Snack

Almonds (25)

Lunch

Spicy Chicken Pitas: This recipe requires 15 minutes of preparation,15 minutes to cook and serves 4.

What's in It

- Extra-virgin olive oil (2 T)

- Salt (to taste)
- Black pepper (to taste)
- Red onion (.25 cups sliced thin)
- Tomato (1 sliced)
- Romaine lettuce (1 cup shredded)
- Whole wheat pitas (4 warmed)
- Lemon juice (2 tsp.)
- Cilantro (1 T chopped)
- Mint (1 T chopped)
- Fat free plain Greek Yogurt (.75 cups)
- Cucumber (1 cup sliced thin)
- Garam masala (1.5 tsp.)
- Chicken breast (1 lb. trimmed)

How's It Made

- Heat your grill to a high/medium temperature and oil the rack as needed.
- Coat the chicken with the garam masala, salt and pepper as needed. Grill each side of the chicken for approximately 5 minutes until the internal temperature reads 165 degree Fahrenheit.
- Remove the chicken from the grill and let it cool for 5 minutes before slicing.
- In a small bowl, combine the pepper, salt, remaining garam masala, lemon juice, cilantro, mint, Greek yogurt and cucumber and mix well.
- Split the pitas and fill them with the onion, tomato, lettuce, yogurt sauce and chicken.

Snack

String cheese (1 piece)

Dinner

Broccoli (2 cups)

Brown rice (1 cup)

Chicken Dijon: This recipe requires 5 minutes of preparation, 10 minutes to cook and makes 2 servings.

What's in It

- Olive oil (1 T)
- Black pepper (.5 tsp.)
- Salt (.5 tsp.)
- Parsley (6 sprigs)
- Dijon mustard (2 tsp.)
- Garlic (1 clove crushed)
- Chicken breast (8 oz. portioned)

How's It Made

- Heat your grill to a medium heat.
- In a small bowl, mix together the pepper, salt, parsley mustard and garlic and combine well.
- Coat the chicken in the mixture.
- Grill the chicken for 5 minutes per side, the chicken's internal temperature should be 165 degrees Fahrenheit.

Day 7

Breakfast

Eggs (2)

Vegetable (1)

Grapefruit (1 medium)

Snack

Protein bar (1)

Lunch

Turkey Tostada: This recipe requires 30 minutes of preparation, 10 minutes to cook and serves 4.

What's in It

- Extra-virgin olive oil (2 tsp.)
- Salt (to taste)
- Black pepper (to taste)
- Monterey Jack cheese (.5 cups)
- Romaine lettuce (1 cup shredded)
- Low fat sour cream (2 T)
- Salsa (.25 cups)
- Avocado (1 pitted)
- Corn tortillas (8)
- Turkey (3 cups shredded, cooked)
- Onion (1 sliced thin)
- Tomatoes (14 oz. diced)
- Jalapeno (1 chopped, seeded)

How's It Made

- Ensure your oven is heated to 375 degrees Fahrenheit. Set your oven racks to the lower and upper thirds.
- Boil the tomatoes using their own canned juice in a saucepan placed on a burner turned to a medium heat. Mix in the onion and let it cook

for 15 minutes before mixing in the turkey and letting it cook for 1.5 minutes.

- Add the oil to both sides of the tortillas and place them on a pair of baking sheets.
- Place the baking sheets in the oven and bake for 5 minutes, turn the sheets and bake for another 5 minutes.
- In a small bowl, smash the avocado and mix in the cilantro, sour cream and salsa and mix well.
- Top the tortillas with avocado, the turkey mix, cheese and lettuce prior to serving.

Snack

Raisins (2 boxes)

Dinner

Brown rice (1 cup)

Edamame and Salmon: This recipe requires 20 minutes of preparation, 8 minutes to cook and makes 4 servings.

What's in It

- Edamame (1.3 cups cooked)
- Black sesame seed (.25 tsp.)
- Honey (2 tsp.)
- Low fat soy sauce (2 tsp.)
- Lime juice (2 tsp.)
- Salmon fillet (24 oz. portioned)
- Black pepper (to taste)
- Salt (to taste)
- Ginger (1 tsp.)
- Extra virgin olive oil (2 tsp.)
- Scallions (2)
- Cilantro leaves (.25 cups packed)

How's It Made

- Ensure your grill is heated to a high/medium heat and is oiled.
- In a bowl, combine the ginger, oil, scallion and cilantro before seasoning as desired.
- Cut a 3-inch slit in the bottom of each fillet and add the mixture to each before seasoning the fish as needed.
- In a small bowl, combine the honey, soy and lime juice.
- Place the fish on the grill and let each side cook for 4 minutes. Top the fish with the lime, soy and honey sauce.

Chapter 7: Week 4

Day 1

Breakfast

      Eggs (3 scrambled)

      Grapefruit (1 large)

Snack

      String Cheese (1)

Lunch

      Chicken Curry Pita (Week 2, Day 1)

Snack

      Fat free Greek yogurt (1 serving)

Dinner

      Side Salad with vinegar/olive oil (2 T)

      Pasta and Spicy Chicken (Week 1, Day 1)

Day 2

Breakfast

      Toast (1 piece)

      Peanut Butter (2 T)

Snack

      Box of raisins (2 small)

Lunch

      Salmon Sammie (Week 2, Day 2)

Snack

      Almonds (25)

Dinner

      Snow peas (2 cups)

      Asian Lettuce Wraps (Week 2, Day 1)

Day 3

Breakfast

      Eggs (2)

      Ham (1 slice)

Snack

      Snap Peas (15)

      Hummus (2 T)

Lunch

      Charred Tomato, Broccoli and Chicken Salad (Week 2, Day 3)

Snack

      1 Banana

Dinner

      Brown Rice (1 cup)

Broccoli (2 cups)

Tofu and Broccoli Stir Fry (Week 2, Day 2)

Day 4

Breakfast

Eggs (2)

Vegetable (1)

Banana (1)

Snack

Baby carrots (30)

Hummus (4 T)

Lunch

Sun Dried Tomato, Corn and Turkey Wrap (Week 2, Day 4)

Snack

Fat free Greek yogurt (1 serving)

Dinner

Broccoli (2 cups)

Brown rice (1 cup)

Chicken Dijon (Week 3, Day 6)

Day 5

Breakfast

      Fat free Greek Yogurt (1 serving)

      Grapefruit (1 large)

Snack

      1 Banana

Lunch

      Crab Roll (Week 2, Day 5)

Snack

      Snap Peas (15)

      Hummus (2 T)

Dinner

      Broccoli (2 cups)

      Brown Rice (1 cup)

      Chicken with Lime and Cilantro (Week 2, Day 4)

Day 6

Breakfast

      Scrambled eggs (3)

      Grapefruit (1 large)

Snack

      Protein bar (1)

Lunch

   White Bean Salad with Chicken (Week 2, Day 6)

Snack

   Almonds (25)

Dinner

   Side Salad with vinegar and olive oil (4 T)

   Sweet Potato Fries (1 serving)

   Veggie Burger with Whole Wheat Bun (Week 1, Day 3)

Day 7

Breakfast

   Eggs (2)

   Vegetable (1)

   String cheese (1)

Snack

   Box of raisins (2 small)

Lunch

   Tarragon chicken salad (Week 2, Day 7)

Snack

   Fat free Greek yogurt (1 serving)

Dinner

Broccoli (2 cups)

Sour and Sweet Chicken and Brown Rice (Week 2, Day 3)

Chapter 8: Week 5

Day 1

Breakfast

      Eggs (3 scrambled)

      Grapefruit (1 large)

Snack

      Fat free Greek yogurt (1 serving)

Lunch

      Turkey Wrap (Week 1, Day 1)

Snack

      Snap Peas (15)

      Hummus (2 T)

Dinner

      Broccoli (2 cups)

      Fettuccine with Peas and Shrimp (Week 3, Day 1)

Day 2

Breakfast

      Toast (1 slice)

      Peanut Butter (2 T)

Snack

Almonds (25)

Lunch

Chicken Sausage with Peppers (Week 1, Day 2)

Snack

Baby carrots (30)

Hummus (4 T)

Dinner

Broccoli (2 cups)

Miso Salmon (Day 2, Week 1)

Day 3

Breakfast

Eggs (2)

Vegetable (1)

Grapefruit (1 large)

Snack

1 Banana

Lunch

White Beans with Pesto and Asparagus (Week 1, Day 3)

Snack

Box of raisins (2 small)

Dinner

Brown rice (1 cup)

Broccoli (2 cups)

Dill Sauce and Salmon (Week 2, Day 5)

Day 4

Breakfast

Ham (1 slice)

Eggs (2)

Grapefruit (1 medium)

Snack

Fat free Greek yogurt (1 serving)

Lunch

Chicken Salad Lettuce Wraps (Week 1, Day 4)

Snack

Baby carrots (30)

Hummus (4 T)

Dinner

Brown rice (1 cup)

Veggie Stir Fry (Week 3, Day 2)

Day 5

Breakfast

       Toast (1 slice)

       Peanut butter (2 T)

       Grapefruit (1 large)

Snack

       Almonds (25)

Lunch

       Lean Soufflé (Week 1, Day 5)

Snack

       Snap Peas (15)

       Hummus (2 T)

Dinner

       Broccoli (2 cups)

       Brown rice (1 cup)

       Snapper and Pesto (Week 1, Day 4)

Day 6

Breakfast

       Eggs (2)

Vegetable (1)

Grapefruit (1 large)

Snack

Fat free Greek yogurt (1 serving)

Lunch

Sesame Tofu, Scallion and Ginger (Week 1, Day 6)

Snack

1 Banana

Dinner

Broccoli (2 cups)

Brown Rice (1 cup)

Poblanos Stuffed with Barley (Week 2, Day 6)

Day 7

Breakfast

Eggs (3 scrambled)

Grapefruit (1 large)

Snack

Box of raisins (2 small)

Lunch

Mango Salsa and Pork Tenderloin (Week 1, Day 7)

Snack

Baby carrots (30)

Hummus (4 T)

Dinner

Side salad with vinegar and olive oil (2 T)

Broccoli (2 cups)

Balsamic chicken (Week 3, Day 3)

Chapter 9: Week 6

Day 1

Breakfast

>Oatmeal (1 serving)

>Grapefruit (1 large)

Snack

>Banana (1)

>Fat free Greek yogurt (1 serving)

Lunch

>Tofu Peanut Wrap (Week 4, Day 1)

Snack

>Box of raisins (2 small)

Dinner

>Snow peas (2 cups)

>Brown rice (1 cup)

>Spinach with Chicken Parmesan (Week 1, Day 5)

Day 2

Breakfast

>Ham (1 slice)

>Eggs (2)

Grapefruit (1 medium)

Snack

Snap Peas (15)

Hummus (2 T)

Lunch

Turkey Lettuce Wrap (Week 3, Day 2)

Snack

Fat free Greek yogurt (1 serving)

Dinner

Side salad with vinegar and olive oil (2 T)

Baja Fish Tacos (Week 2, Day 7)

Day 3

Breakfast

Toast (1 slice)

Peanut butter (2 T)

Grapefruit (1 medium)

Snack

Almonds (25)

Lunch

Cobb Salad (Week 3, Day 3)

Snack

       Baby carrots (30)

       Hummus (4 T)

Dinner

       Broccoli (2 cups)

       Brown rice (1 cup)

       Swai Fillet (Week 3, Day 4)

Day 4

Breakfast

       Eggs (3 scrambled)

       Grapefruit (1 large)

Snack

       1 Banana

Lunch

       Tuna Panini (Week 3, Day 4)

Snack

       Cherry Tomatoes (10)

       Hummus (2 T)

Dinner

       Broccoli (2 cups)

Brown rice (1 cup)

Lemon Chicken with Dill (Week 1, Day 6)

Day 5

Breakfast

Eggs (2)

Vegetable (1)

Grapefruit (1 medium)

Snack

Box of raisins (2 small)

Lunch

Red Lentil Curry Soup (Week 3, Day 5)

Snack

Baby carrots (30)

Hummus (4 T)

Dinner

Side salad with vinegar and olive oil (2 T)

Bean Quesadilla (Week 3, Day 5)

Day 6

Breakfast

Eggs (3 scrambled)

Grapefruit (1 large)

Snack

Almonds (25)

Banana (1)

Lunch

Spicy Chicken Pitas (Week 3, Day 6)

Snack

Snap Peas (15)

Hummus (2 T)

Dinner

Broccoli (2 cups)

Chicken Marengo and Penne (Week 1, Day 7)

Day 7

Breakfast

Toast (1 piece)

Peanut Butter (2 T)

Snack

Almonds (25)

Lunch

Turkey Tostada (Week 3, Day 7)

Snack

Fat free Greek yogurt (1 serving)

Almonds (25)

Dinner

Brown rice (1 cup)

Edamame and Salmon (Week 3, Day 7)

Conclusion

Thank you again for downloading this book! I hope this book was able to help you to learn everything you need to in order to take advantage of all of the opportunities that sticking with a lean lifestyle offers. It is important to keep up the good work now that you are at the end of your 6-week struggle. Remember how hard you had to fight to get here and don't let it all go to waste. Being lean is a journey, not a destination, and your journey is just beginning.

The next step is to stop reading already and use the recipes you have learned as a blueprint for future culinary adventures. Remember to stick with clean ingredients as strictly as possible and you can't go wrong. Happy eating!

Finally, if you enjoyed this book, then I'd like to ask you for a favor, would you be kind enough to leave a review for this book on Amazon? It'd be greatly appreciated!

Free Bonus!

As promised, here is your free Low-Carb Cookbook! Just visit the link below to download!

http://www.xcensionpublishing.com/LowCarbCookbookBC.pdf

www.ingramcontent.com/pod-product-compliance
Lightning Source LLC
Chambersburg PA
CBHW060238290526
45789CB00001B/106